Color Atlas of Cutaneous Infections

Color Atlas of Cutaneous Infections

Lawrence Charles Parish, M.D.

Clinical Professor of Dermatology
Director, Jefferson Center for International Dermatology
Jefferson Medical College
Thomas Jefferson University
Philadelphia, Pennsylvania
Adjunct Professor of Comparative Dermatology
University of Pennsylvania School of Veterinary Medicine
Philadelphia, Pennsylvania
Visiting Professor of Dermatology
Yonsei University College of Medicine
Seoul, Korea
Visiting Professor of Dermatology and Venereology
Zagazig University
Zagazig, Egypt

Joseph A. Witkowski, M.D.

Clinical Professor of Dermatology
University of Pennsylvania School of Medicine
Philadelphia, Pennsylvania
Professor of Dermatology
Pennsylvania College of Podiatric Medicine
Philadelphia, Pennsylvania

Snejina Vassileva, M.D., Ph.D.

Assistant Professor of Dermatology
Sofia Faculty of Medicine
Sofia, Bulgaria

Blackwell
Science

Blackwell Science

Editorial Offices: 238 Main Street, Cambridge, Massachusetts 02142, USA
Osney Mead, Oxford OX2 0EL, England
25 John Street, London WC1N 2BL, England
23 Ainslie Place, Edinburgh EH3 6AJ, Scotland
54 University Street, Carlton, Victoria 3053, Australia
Arnette Blackwell SA, 1 rue de Lille, 75007 Paris, France
Blackwell Wissenschafts-Verlag GmbH, Kurfürstendamm 57, 10707 Berlin, Germany
Feldgasse 13, A-1238 Vienna, Austria

Distributors:

North America
Blackwell Science, Inc.
238 Main Street, Cambridge, Massachusetts 02142
(Telephone orders: 800-215-1000 or 617-876-7000)

Australia
Blackwell Science Pty, Ltd.
54 University Street, Carlton, Victoria 3053
(Telephone orders: 03-347-5552)

Outside North America and Australia
Blackwell Science, Ltd.
c/o Marston Book Services, Ltd., P.O. Box 87, Oxford OX2 0DT, England
(Telephone orders: 44-1865-791155)

Acquisitions: Victoria Reeders
Development: Coleen Traynor
Production: A. Maria Hight and Paula Card Higginson
Manufacturing: Kathleen Grimes
Designed and composed: Leslie Haimes, Swampscott, MA
Printed and bound by G. Canale & C., Turin, Italy

95 96 97 98 5 4 3 2 1

Library of Congress Cataloging in Publication Data
Parish, Lawrence Charles.
Color atlas of cutaneous infections/Lawrence Charles Parish, Joseph A. Witkowski, Snejina Vassileva.
p. cm.
Includes bibliographical reference and index.
ISBN 0-86542-435-7
1. Skin—Infections—Atlases. I. Witkowski, Joseph A.
II. Vassileva, Snejina. III. Title
RL201.P37 1995
616.5'0022'2—dc20 94-39441
CIP

To the memory of

Orlando Cañizares, M.D.

who first conceived of this book

Table of Contents

Preface

Infections and infestations have always played a major role in the study of diseases of the skin structure. Sometimes, they are the primary dermatologic entity, and at other times they complicate a preexisting dermatitis. Still, at other times, the skin becomes the reflection of a localized or systemic infection or infestation in another organ system.

HISTORICAL ASPECTS

The concept of skin disease due to microscopic organisms was not always so readily accepted. Erasmus Wilson (1809–1884), the distinguished London surgeon, offered a prize to anyone who could prove that fungi had no role in the causation of ringworm (Figure 1). In discussing favus, Wilson wrote in his popular nineteenth-century textbook (1):

> ...the absence of the cellated shafts is an additional ground of argument against the vegetable theory. It is perfectly consistent with the pathology of abnormal nutrition, that the hair-granules should become enlarged and increase in number by proliferation, and thus be the cause of the subsequent changes taking place in the hair. But the hypothesis of vegetable growth within the substance of the hair is to us impossible to comprehend.

Yet Louis Duhring (1845–1913), the pathfinder for dermatology, published his first paper on the subject of alopecia areata, demonstrating that this entity was not due to a fungal infection (2). He also recognized that dermatophyte infections were caused by fungi (Figure 2).

If the pendulum was to swing so far by then end of the nineteenth-century that every disease had its own bacteria (3), then it is difficult to grasp how the professor of hygiene at the University of Pennsylvania, Joseph G. Richardson (1836–1886) prepared a lecture on the germ theory in which he pled for its acceptance some two decades after its current inception (4):

> ...the Germ Theory of Disease, which was propounded by the celebrated Linnaues more than a century ago, but has since been somewhat modified by its successive advocates, professes to account for the phenomena of small-pox, typhoid fever, yellow fever, relapsing fever, measles, scarlatina, diphtheria, chicken-pox, erysipelas, etc., by attributing them to the more or less mechanical irritation and other disturbances set up by masses of spores and mycelial threads developing in the blood and in the affected tissues.

PURPOSE

The idea of this atlas was first suggested by the late Orlando Cañizares (1910–1992) of New York, pioneer leader in the field of tropical dermatology (5,6). Cañizares had seen an atlas of cutaneous infections and believed that a much better volume could be created. Unfortunately, he was unable to embark on the project, but his idea became the genesis for this book and to him we have proferred the dedication.

An atlas is meant to be an illustrated text with emphasis on pictures. We have prepared previous color atlases (7–9), but this project presented new challenges. What diseases would be important to the American and European practitioner? If we included only typical types of infection, then there may be no purpose in developing this book. Similarly, if we emphasized the exotic or the tropical varieties of diseases, we would defeat our purpose. Thus, some diseases are included to set the stage for a chapter; while others, albeit rare or strange, are incorporated for their significant didactic value.

We have limited the discussions of various entities, as this volume is not intended to be encyclopedic. Occasionally, variations have been included to to emphasize the versatility of morphology. Some diseases have been omitted, not necessarily because they may not be seen in a busy practice, but because appropriate pictures could not be located. The microbiology has not been illustrated, and the reader in search of such pictorial assistance is referred to an excellent volume, Atlas of Medical Microbiology (10).

Although the title of this book indicates our concern with infections, we have liberally defined the word and included several infections. Descriptive text and suggested readings are provided. Though it may be worth a thousand words, a picture is not useful without some definition of the cutaneous entity being depicted.

ACKNOWLEDGMENTS

We acknowledge with deep appreciation all those physicians who graciously have allowed us to use their slides. Without their contributions, we would not have been able to complete this task. We also wish to thank the staff of Blackwell Science for their continuing efforts in producing this book and Dr. Hirak B. Routh and Ms. Carmela Ciferni, Philadelphia, who provided editorial assistance.

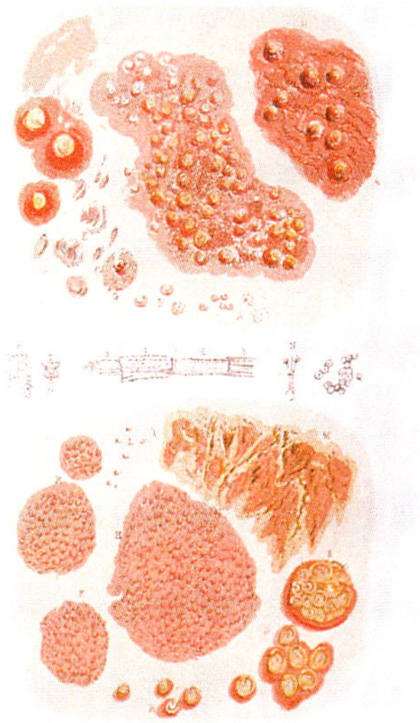

Figure 1
Acne, sycosis, trichosis, favus. Most of this plate shows the scales and crusts taken from dermatophyte infections. Wilson did not believe that there was a cause and effect relationship between ringworm and fungi. (Reproduced from Wison E. Diseases of the skin. Philadelphia: Henry C. Lea, 1863: plate xiv.)

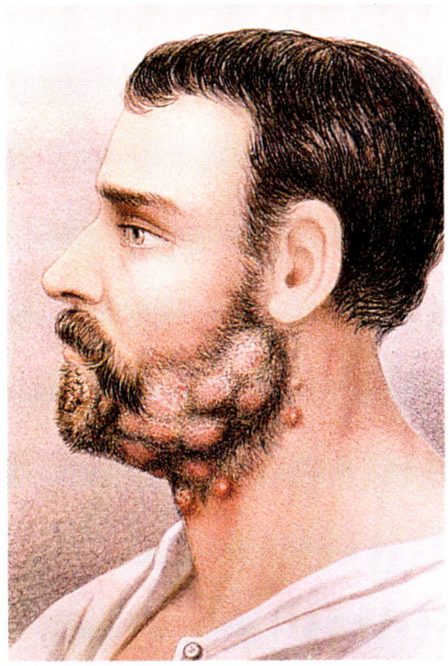

Figure 2
Tinea sycosis. Duhring attributes the cause to the presence and growth of the trichophyton fungus within the follicle and hair. (Reproduced from Duhring LA. Atlas of skin diseases. Philadelphia: JB Lippincott, 1876:plate s.)

References

1. Wilson E. Diseases of the Skin: a system of cutaneous medicine. Philadelphia: Henry C. Lea, 1868:642–648.

2. Duhring LA. Pathology of alopecia areata. Am J Med Sci 1870;60:122–126.

3. Castiglioni A. A history of medicine. New York: Alfred A. Knopf, 1947:817–819.

4. Richardson JG. The germ theory of disease and its present bearing upon public and personal hygiene. (Read before the Philadelphia Social Sciences Association, Oct 17, 1878.) Philadelphia: E. Stern & Co., 1878:1–14. (Reprinted from Penn Monthly, Nov 1878.)

5. Cipollaro VA. Orlando Cañizares, MD (1910–1992) — as I remember him. Int J Dermatol 1992;31:666-667.

6. Domínguez-Soto L. Orlando Cañizares and Latin American dermatology. Int J Dermatol 1992;31:667–668.

7. Parish LC, Seghal VN, Buntin DM. Color atlas of sexually transmitted diseases. New York: Igaku-Shoin, 1991:1–173.

8. Parish LC, Kauh YC, Luscombe HA. Color atlas of difficult diagnoses in dermatology. New York: Igaku-Shoin, 1993:1–144.

9. Witkowski JA, Lemont HA. Color atlas of the lower extremities. New York: Igaku-Shoin, 1993.

10. Mangelschots E, Lontie M, Vandepitte J. Atlas of medical microbiology. Belgium: Acco, 1990:1–126.

Color Atlas of Cutaneous Infections

BACTERIA

Bacteria are unicellular organisms with rigid walls. They usually reproduce asexually through binary fission. These "germs" are viewed best microscopically through the oil-immersion lens with the aid of gram staining. Gram-positive bacteria that retain the methyl violet stain are seen as deep violet, whereas gram-negative bacteria take up the counterstain carbol fuchsin and appear pink. By definition, *aerobic bacteria* require oxygen and *anaerobic bacteria* grow better in an oxygen deprived atmosphere.

PYOGENIC INFECTIONS

The pyogenic infections are the most common of the many bacterial infections involving the skin. They were originally termed pyogenic because of their pus producing capabilities, but the classification by contemporary standards is purely arbitrary.

ETIOLOGY

Pyogenic infections are caused predominantly by *Staphylococcus aureus* and *ß-hemolytic Streptococcus*, Group A. Several other bacteria have been identified as having similar pathogenic qualities for producing skin and skin structure infection (Table 1).

Table 1 Bacteria Found on the Skin

Normal flora	Common pathogens	Uncommon pathogens
aerobic		
Staphylococcus epidermidis	*Staphylococcus aureus*	Actinetobacter sp
Staphylococcus saprophyticus	*Staphylococcus epidermidis*	Enterobacter sp
Micrococcus	*ß hemolytic Streptococcus*,GpA	*Streptococcus faecalis*
Corynebacterium	*Escherichia coli*	Klebsiella sp
Brevibacterium	*Morganella morganii*	*Providencia stuartii*
	Proteus mirabilis	*Serratia marcescens*
	Proteus vulgaris	*Streptococcus agalactiae*
	Pseudomonas aeruginosa	*ß hemolytic Streptococcus,* Gp B, C, and G
anaerobic		
Propionibacterium acnes	*Bacteroides fragilis*	
Propionibacterium avidum	*Clostridium perfringens*	

CLINICAL PRESENTATION

These infections may be classified as primary (the infection consists of lesions that are not associated with another cutaneous malady or a systemic infection); secondary (the infection is secondary to an underlying and/or preexisting dermatitis); or tertiary (the cutaneous findings are secondary to a systemic infection).

PRIMARY INFECTIONS (TABLE 2):

Table 2 Primary Infections According to Anatomical Considerations

Epidermal	Dermal	Circumscribed	Appendageal
impetigo	cellulitis	abscess	carbuncle
ecthyma	erysipelas	paronychia	folliculitis
	lymphangitis		furuncle
	pyoderma		

Abscess A red, tender, dome-shaped lesion that develops a fluctuant center (Figure 1).

Carbuncle A tense, indurated, red lesion that is painful and has several pustular openings. It involves several hair follicles and is usually found on the neck (Figure 2).

Cellulitis Induration extending from the dermis to the subcutaneous tissue, with heat, redness, induration, and tenderness. There may be accompanying fever and chills. The organism gains entry through an opening or break in the skin (Figure 3a). Chronic cellulitis leads to elephantiasis, which generally is nonreversible (Figure 3b).

Ecthyma An erythematous, indurated, tender lesion, covered by a hemorrhagic crust. It might be considered as a deeper form of impetigo (Figure 4).

Erysipelas A dermal infection, most often due to streptococci, that has sudden onset. There is redness, swelling, and sharp borders. Vesicles and bullae may occur on the surface. It is usually accompanied by pain and tenseness of the tissue (Figure 5).

Folliculitis A superficial infection of the hair follicle, characterized by follicular, erythematous papules or pustules. Crusting, pruritus, tenderness, and pain may ensue (Figures 6a,b). Various forms include pseudofolliculitis barbae (Figure 6c), perifolliculitis capitis abscendens et suffodiens (Figure 6d), and pseudomonas folliculitis or "hot tub dermatitis" (Figure 6e).

Furuncle Also called a *boil,* this lesion resembles the carbuncle except for having one pustular opening. Many discrete furuncles create the condition termed *furunculosis.* Should adjacent furuncles coalesce, they create a carbuncle (Figure 7).

Lymphangitis An erythematous streak that follows the lymphatics. Many times, the infectious process produces tenderness (Figure 8).

Paronychia An inflammatory process of the tissue surrounding the nail. The pathogens are usually staphylococci, but streptococci, *Pseudomonas aeruginosa*, and *Candida albicans* are often involved. The process may occur as a result of moisture creating edema and fissuring, resulting in separation of the eponychium from the nail plate. This permits the pathogen to penetrate into the nail fold. When the tissue dries out, the pathogens become loculated (Figure 9a,b).

Pyoderma or impetigo A process characterized by erythema, crusting, and even bullous formation, sometimes associated with pruritus, tenderness, and pain. The terms *impetigo* and *pyoderma* are used interchangeably, although the former denotes an infection in the epidermis and the latter a process extending through the dermis into the subcutaneous tissue. While staphylococci are usually responsible for the bullous type and streptococci for the vesicular to yellow crusted variety, both types of organisms can produce the yellow crusted variety of infections (Figures 10a,b).

Bullous impetigo may be considered a localized form of staphylococcal scalded skin syndrome (SSSS), caused by *S. aureus*, phage group II, mostly phage type 71. Whereas in bullous impetigo the exotoxin is produced in the bullous lesions, in SSSS the toxin is produced in the umbilical stump, conjunctivae, external ears, or nares, from which it is disseminated (Figure 10c).

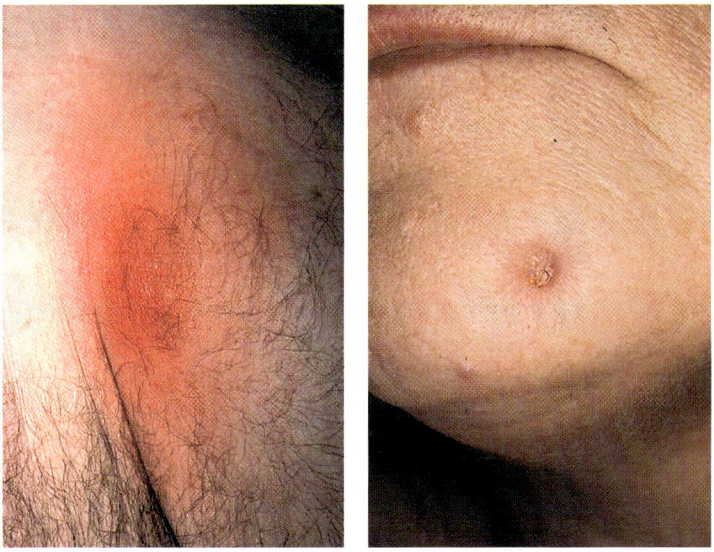

a b

Figure 1
An abscess is a walled-off lesion that may be firm and tender. (a) This lesion on the buttocks required incision and drainage, while (b) the lesion on the cheek, an apical root abscess, reflects poor dental hygiene leading to caries formation in the sinus tract.

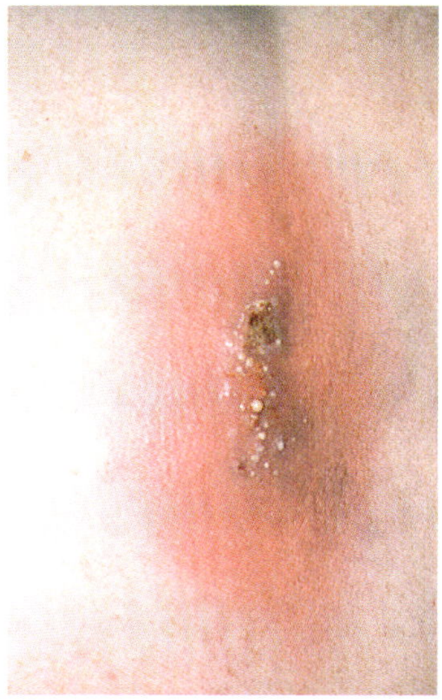

Figure 2
A carbuncle is characterized by multiple pustular openings. There is intense perilesional inflammation.

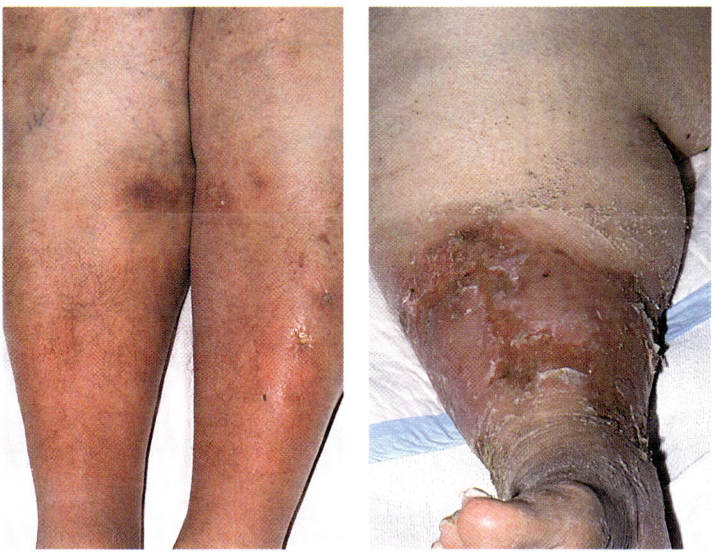

a b

Figure 3
Cellulitis often occurs on the legs. (a) The legs show swelling, redness, and induration, which are more noticeable on the left leg. The purulent area may represent the portal of entry. (b) Chronic infection can lead to permanent swelling, induration, and fibrosis (i.e., elephantiasis).

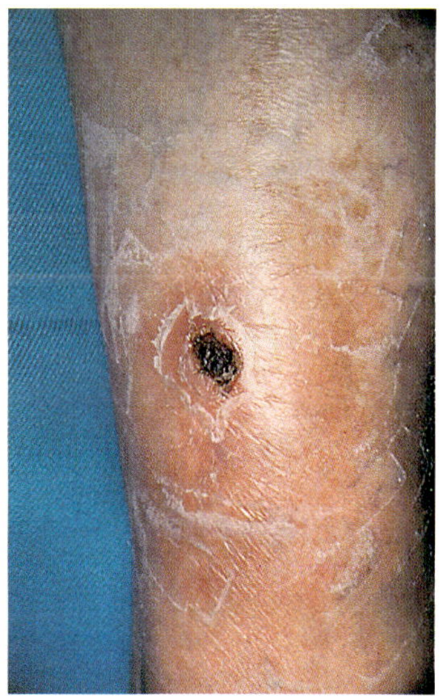

Figure 4
In ecthyma, the infectious process extends into the subcutaneous tissue and causes a necrotic crust and erythema.

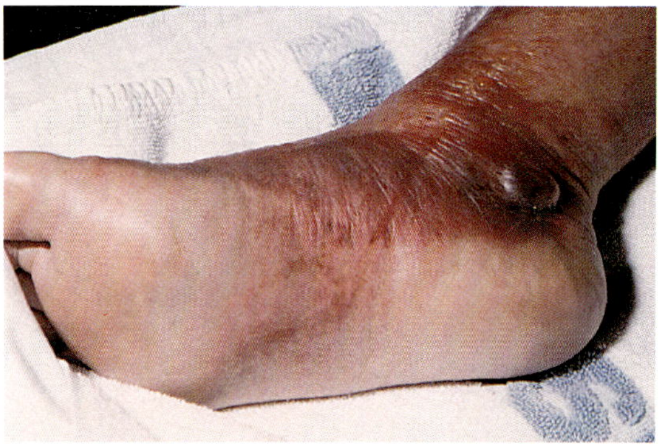

Figure 5
The pathogen, causing the extensive erysipelas in this patient's leg, was *ß-hemolytic streptococcus*, Group A. Notice the sharp borders.

Figure 6
Folliculitis can range from a minor condition to a destructive process. (a) This patient developed follicular papules and pustules on the back after long-term application of topical steroids. (b) The follicular process in the axilla was precipitated by *S. aureus* and is superimposed on an underlying hidradenitis suppurativa. (c) Folliculitis on the beard area is called pseudofolliculitis barbae. (d) Perifolliculitis capitis abscendens et suffodiens (dissecting cellulitis) is a recurrent and scarring problem of the scalp, found more often in black people. (e) Pseudomonas folliculitis developed in this patient following use of the family hot tub. Other members of the family were similarly affected. (Courtesy of Ricardo M. Mandojana, MD, Maryville, TN.)

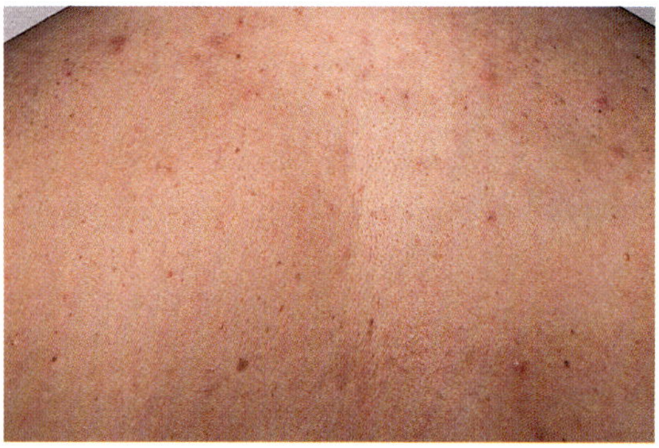

a

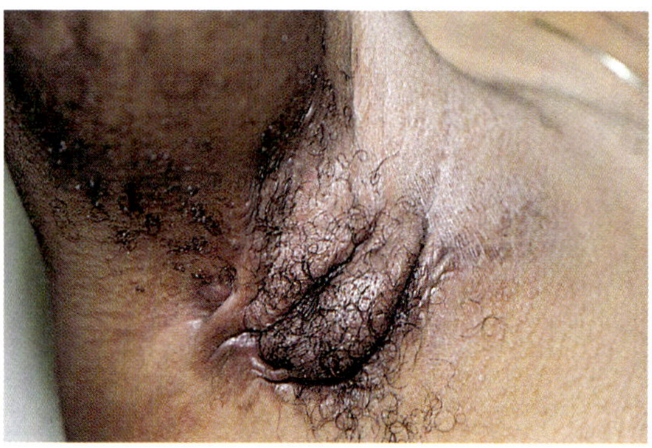

b

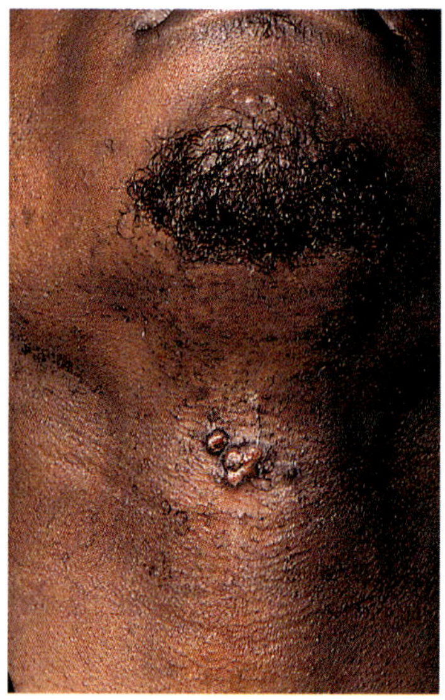

c

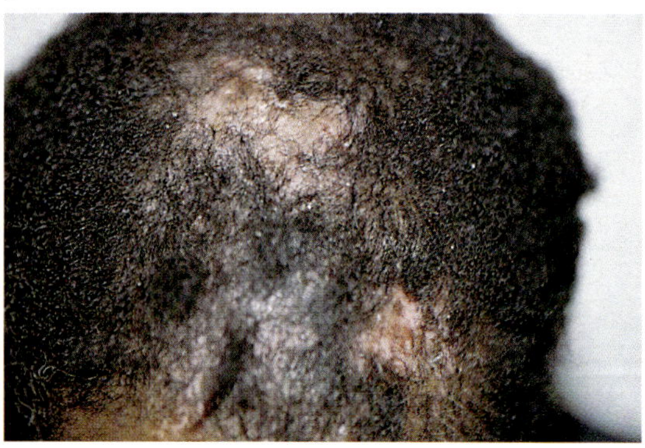

d

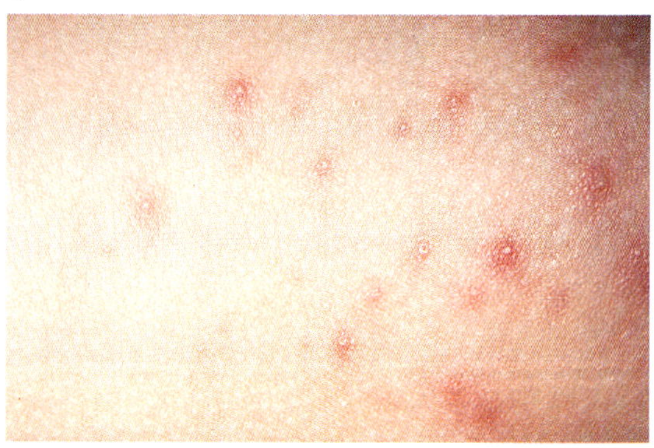

e

Figure 7
A furuncle has a single pustular opening.

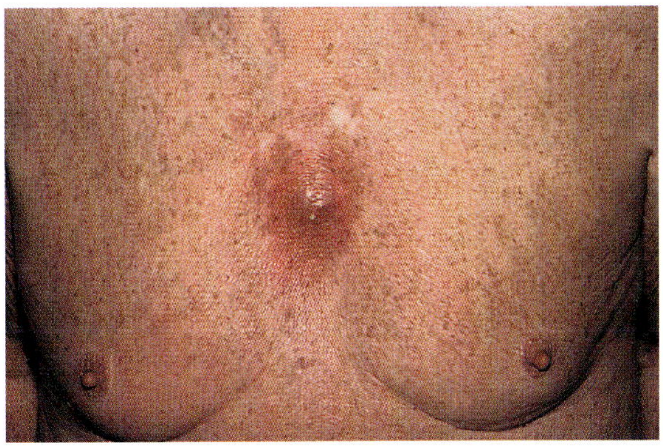

Figure 8
Lymphangitis is very difficult to discern, unless the red streak is seen in appropriate light. The ascending infection is shown on the inner aspect of the arm. (Courtesy of Antar Padilha-Gonçalves, MD, Rio de Janeiro, Brazil.)

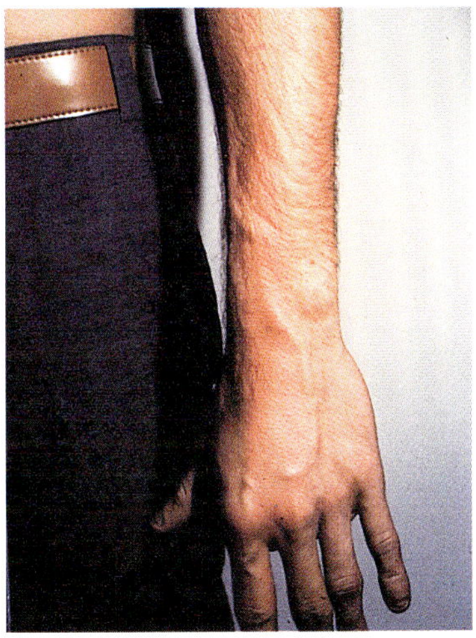

Figure 9
(a) This patient developed an acute paronychia due to housework. It is depicted with swelling, erythema, and bullous formation surrounding the nail. (b) In chronic paronychia, there is less edema and redness at the proximal nail fold. The nails show greenish discoloration due to *P. aeruginosa* infection.

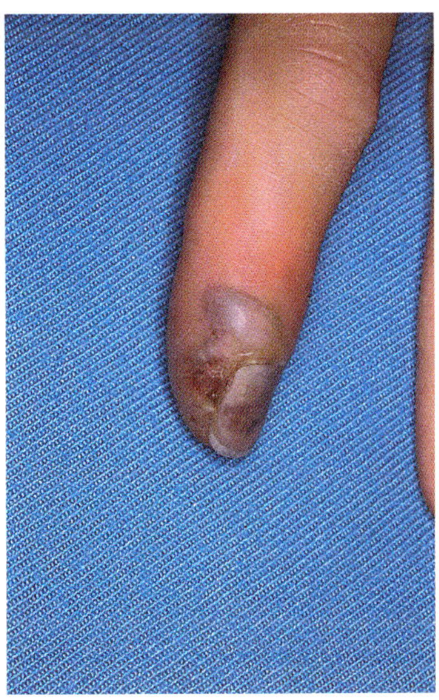

a

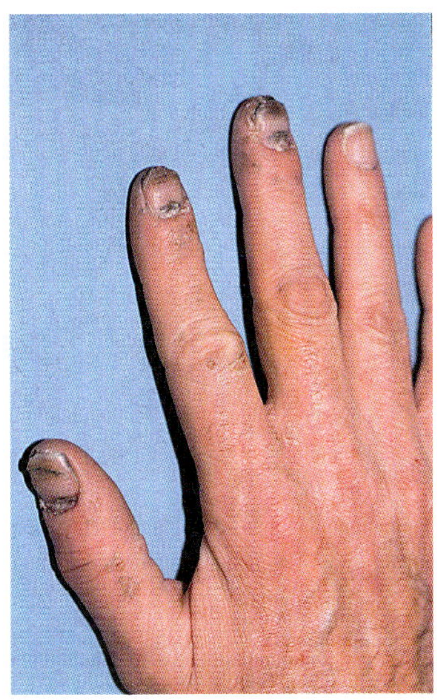

b

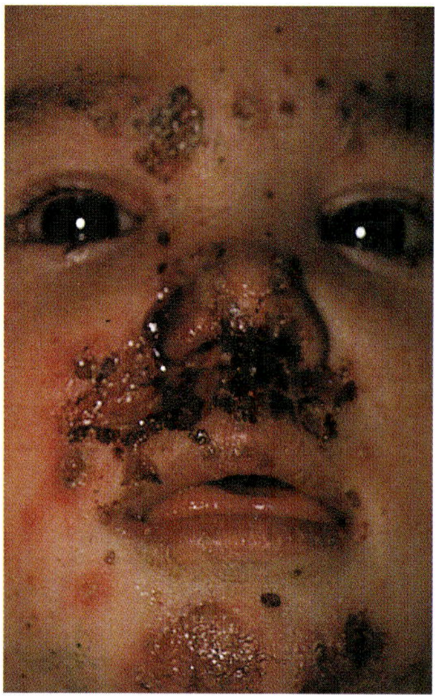

a

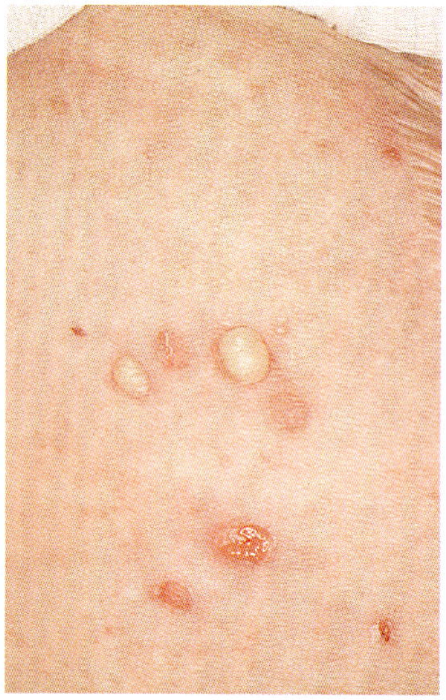

b

Figure 10
(a) Pyoderma often accompanies an upper respiratory tract viral infection, as it did in this child. *ß-hemolytic Streptococcus*, Group A was cultured from his lesion. (b) Yellowish crusts and pustules, due to both staphylococci and streptococci, occurred in this man. (Courtesy of Antar Padilha-Gonçalves, MD, Rio de Janeiro, Brazil.) (c) This child had bullous impetigo due to staphylococci.

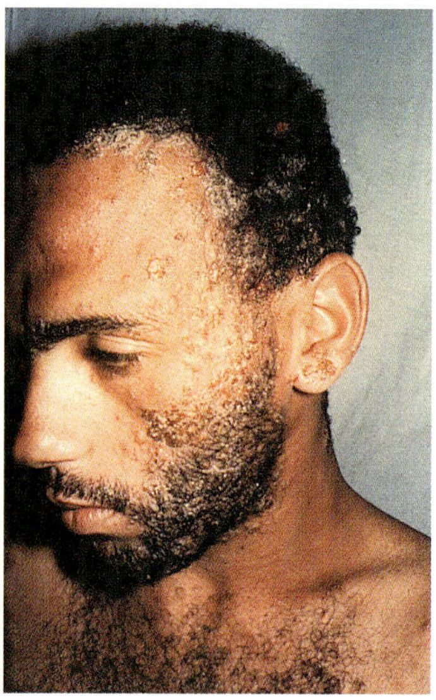

c

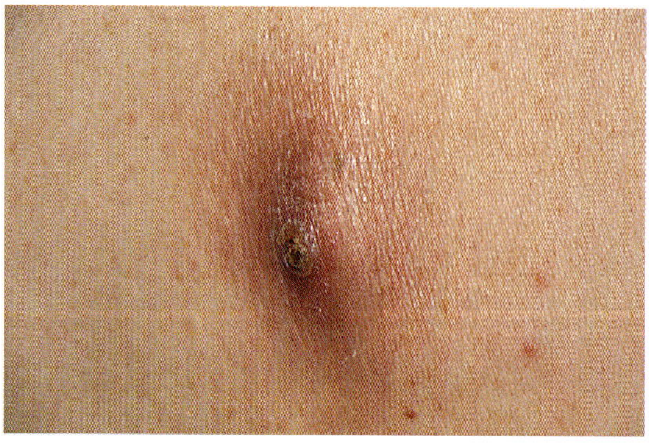

Figure 11
An epidermoid cyst can suddenly become infected, creating pain and tenderness.

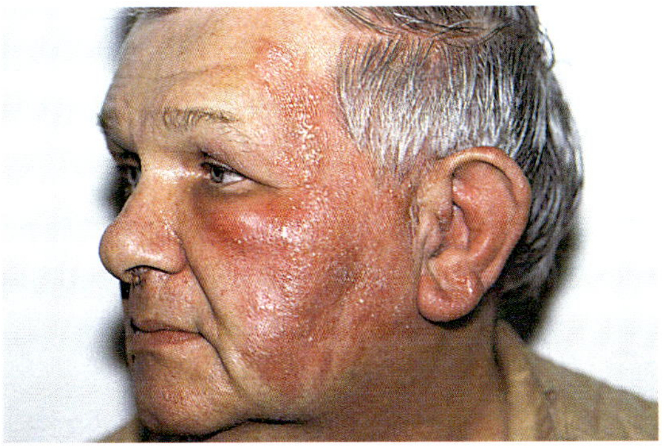

a

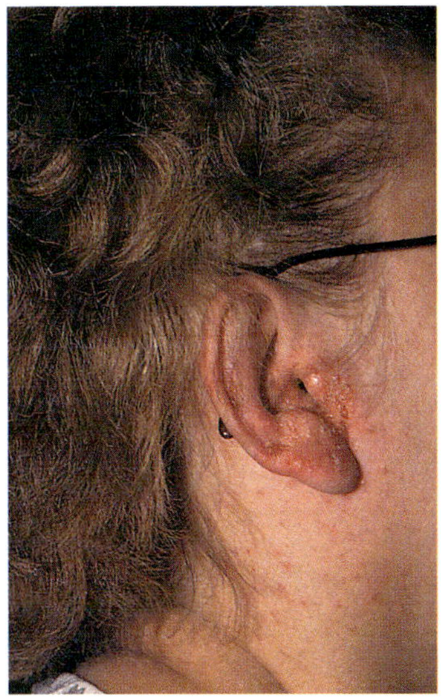

b

Figure 12
(a) Contact dermatitis can easily become secondarily infected. (b) Infectious eczematoid dermatitis reflects a local reaction to pus coming from a site of infection.

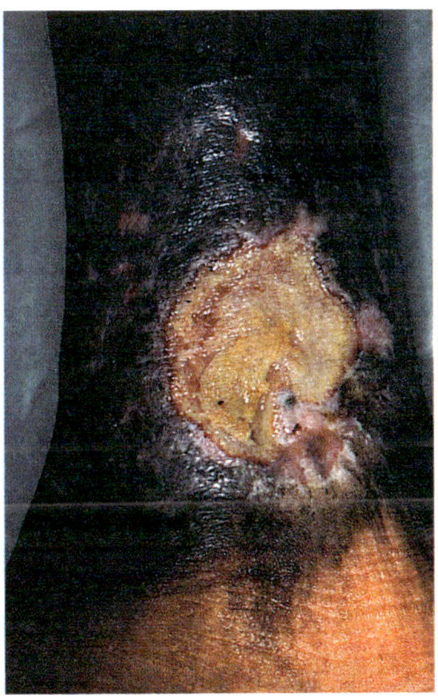

a

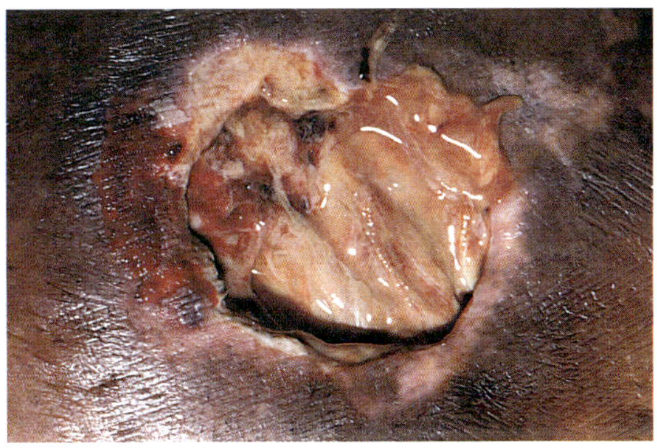

b

Figure 13
(a) This patient with sickle cell anemia often developed secondary infection in her leg ulcer. (b) A decubitus ulcer is prone to infection. This patient's ulcer contained *E. coli* and *P. aeruginosa*.

Figure 14
This infection at a surgical site developed several days after a lesion was excised.

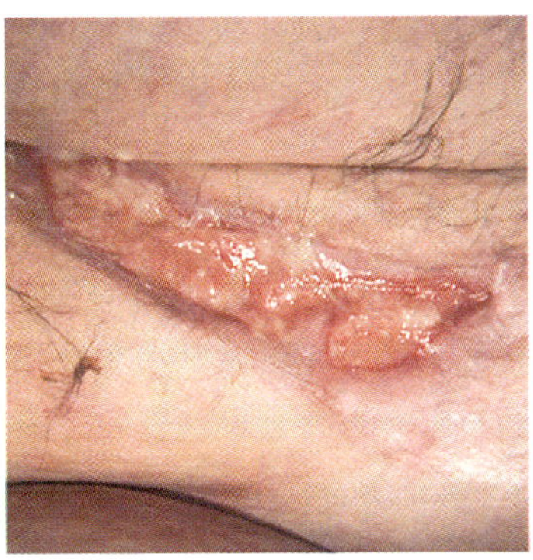

Secondary Infections:

Infected cyst Also called a wen, this is a closed sac lined by epidermally or adnexally developed epithelium. There may be erythema, tenderness, pain, inflammation, and pus. Ruptured cysts are often misdiagnosed as being infected (Figure 11).

Infected dermatitis Already damaged skin, being further aggravated. Although bacteria colonize the dermatitic skin created by atopy and contactants, only sometimes do the organisms become pathogenic enough to create oozing, redness, crusting, and inflammation. Pain and tenderness may then be added to the symptom of itching (Figures 12a,b).

Infected ulcer Ulcers of various denominations, ranging from stasis ulcers to decubitus ulcers, that become secondarily infected with resulting redness, induration of the surrounding skin, and crusting (Figures 13 a,b).

Infected wound A traumatic or surgical defect that is often inflamed. The addition of pathogenic bacteria may be silent or intensify the redness, heat, and crusting, even leading to ulceration (Figure 14).

Tertiary Infections:

Kawasaki Disease also called *mucocutaneous lymph node syndrome*, is a multisystem vasculitis that is the most common cause of acquired cardiac disease in children. An infectious agent that is increasingly being implicated as the causative organism is the toxic shock syndrome toxin-secreting *S. aureus*. Streptococci and *Yersinia pseudotuberculosis*, as well as several viruses and rickettsiae, have also been hypothesed as the pathogens.

The disease is characterized by cutaneous and mucosal erythema, and edema of the lips. Oropharyngeal, palmar, and plantar erythema may also be observed. Later, there may be desquamation (Figure 15a). This polymorphous exanthem may be morbilliform, scarlatiniform, urticarial, macular, or papular (Figure 15b). There is fever, accompanied by bilateral conjunctivitis and cervical lymphadenopathy. A perineal maculopapular eruption, followed by desquamation, develops in almost two-thirds of the patients.

It often begins with an antibiotic-resistant fever, lasting at least 5 days but can continue up to 2 weeks. During the next few weeks, nausea and vomiting, diarrhea, sterile pyuria, and arthritis or arthralgia occur. Cardiac abnormalities include murmurs, arrhythmias, and even aneurysm and thrombosis formation. By approximately 4 weeks, there may be resolution of the signs and symptoms. Within 40 days to 4 years of the onset of the disease, myocardial fibrosis and endocardial fibroelastosis may develop.

Staphylococcal Scalded Skin Syndrome (SSSS), also known as *Ritter's disease*, is a diffuse exfoliating erythroderma caused by *S. aureus*, often phage type 71, and the exotoxins. The initial sign of this septicemia is an erythema that begins on the face, flexures, and pressure points and rapidly spreads to involve the rest of the body. Within a few days, the skin peels off in sheets. SSSS is only rarely fatal and often resembles a second-degree burn.

A drug-induced form, which is difficult to differentiate, is called *toxic epidermal necrolysis* (TEN) (Figure 16a). TEN involves the mucous membranes and afflicts the subepidermis with vacuolization and necrosis of basal cells. While SSSS is predominantly found in children, TEN is more likely to occur in adults. SSSS in children was formerly called *Ritter von Rittershain disease* (Figure 16b).

ß-hemolytic Streptococcus, Group A produces pyrogenic exotoxin A which causes a strep-induced toxic shock syndrome. In addition to the presence of the so-called strawberry tongue, erythematous desquamation may begin within 1 to 2 weeks of the onset of the exanthem.

Scarlet Fever, or scarlatina, begins 2 to 5 days after infection with *ß-hemolytic Streptococcus*, Group A, and rarely with *S. aureus*. Pharyngitis is accompanied by headache, fever, and vomiting. The streptococci produce erythrogenic toxins, which cause punctate erythema. The skin becomes red and the erythema confluent on the upper aspects of the trunk and spreads to involve the extremities and face (Figure 17a). The eruption is more noticeable in the flexural areas, where the linear distribution of petechiae are called Pastia's lines. The pharynx turns a beefy red and by the second day, the whitish coating of the tongue peels, leaving redness with edematous papillae (strawberry or scarlatina tongue) (Figure 17b). When the erythema and other signs begin to regress, the patient desquamates extensively, the sheets of skin peeling initially from the face.

Gonorrhea is caused by *Neisseria gonorrhoeae*. The bacteria usually infect the reproductive tract. In men, a purulent penile discharge occurs 2 to 5 days after exposure (Figure 18a), whereas in women the cervicitis and salpingitis may not be as symptomatic. Pharyngeal and anorectal infections are also prevalent.

Although disseminated gonococcal infection is rare, it involves fever, chills, arthralgia, and arthritis (Figure 18b). The cutaneous lesions may begin as red macules that become hemorrhagic pustules on the palms (Figure 18c), distal parts, or extremities, hemorrhagic vesicles or papules with central necrosis. Lesions are usually sparse and painful.

Purpura Fulminans is a severe coagulopathy resulting from sepsis most often due to *Neisseria meningitidis* (Figure 19a,b) or *Streptococcus pneumoniae* (Figure 19c), as well as the varicella-zoster virus. There is a release of endotoxins from the bloodstream that leads to activated coagulation and possible microscopic thrombosis of the adrenal glands. Purpura of the skin and mucous membranes are also characteristic of disseminated intravascular coagulopathy. When the adrenal glands are involved, the condition is termed the *Waterhouse-Friderichsen syndrome.*

Typhoid Fever is caused by *Salmonella typhi*, a gram-negative rod, spread through fecal contamination. The organisms create disease within 6 to 12 days after infection. Through hematogenous spread, it causes bacteremia, high fever, chills, abdominal pain, and severe headache. There may be constipation and paralytic ileus or diarrhea. Within the first few days of the disease, rose spots may appear on the trunk (Figure 20).

Ecthyma Gangrenosum is usually a specific finding of *P. aeruginosa septicemia*, although staphylococci and *Klebsiella* species have been implicated. *P. aeruginosa* enters the body through a defect in the skin such as a decubitus ulcer, thermal burn, surgical wound, or gangrenous area or even through otitis externa. Maceration and occlusion of the original problem contributes to the spread of the bacterium, particularly in debilitated or immunosuppressed patients. Lesions most often are found in the groin, axillae, or extremities. They begin as abnormal necrotic vesicles that become

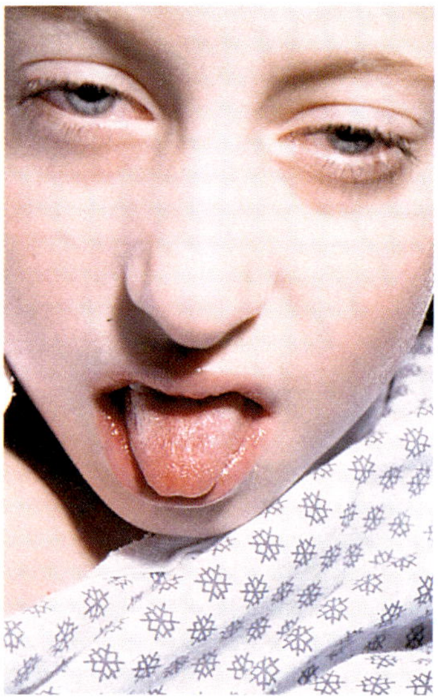

a

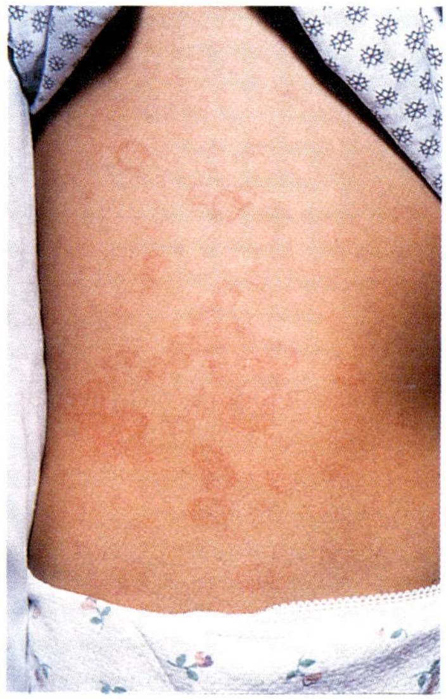

b

Figure 15
Kawasaki disease is manifested by (a) redness and fissuring of the lips with glossal erythema and injection of the bulbar conjunctiva. (b) The patient also has an erythematous eruption consisting of annular lesions that had been preceded by urticaria. (Courtesy of Burke Cuhna, MD, Mineola, NY.)

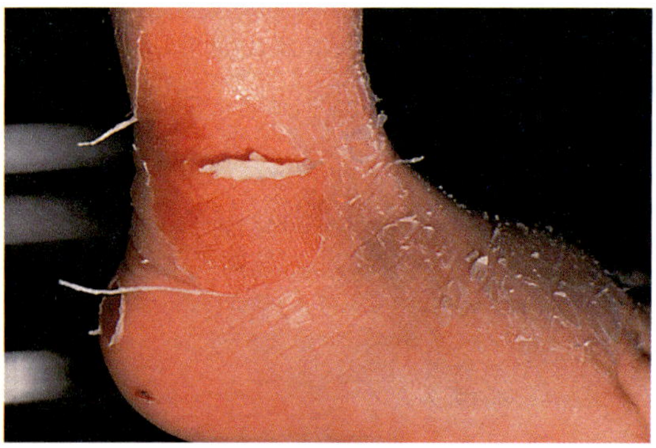

a

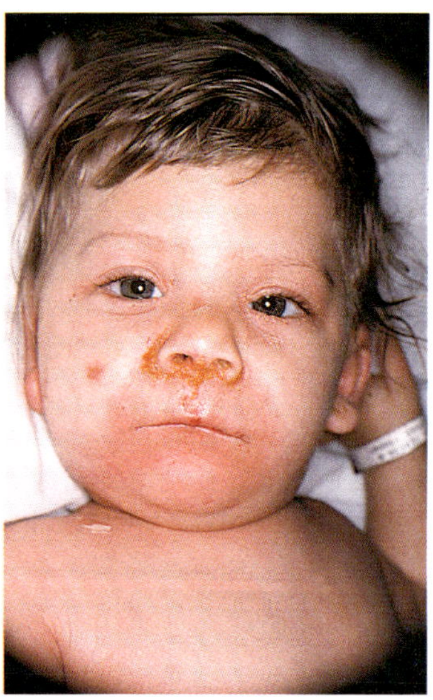

b

Figure 16
Staphylococcal scalded skin syndrome is characterized by erythema and massive desquamation. It is less common (a) in adults than (b) in children.

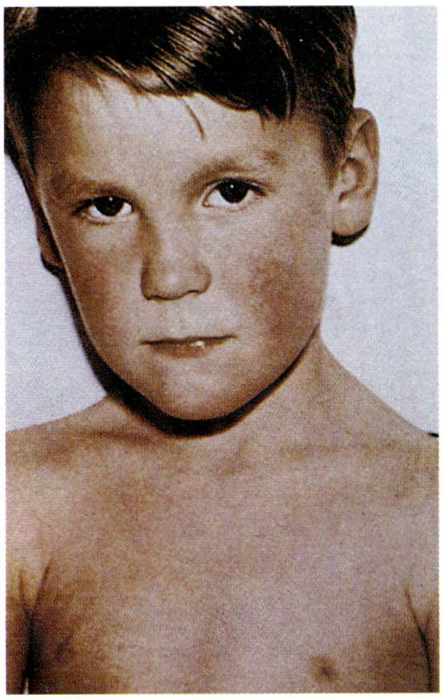

a

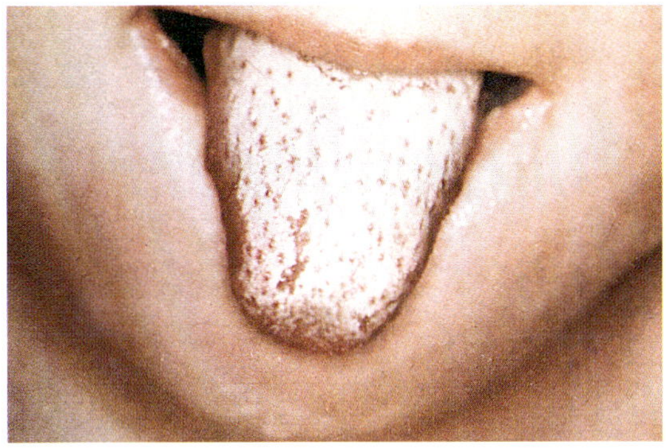

b

Figure 17
Scarlet fever is often recognized by (a) the circumoral palor and facial flushing followed by desquamation, while (b) the tongue is white with reddish papillae giving the appearance of a strawberry. (Courtesy of Sebastião Sampãio, MD, São Paulo, Brazil.)

Figure 18
Gonorrhea is considered the cause of (a) the purulent urethral disease (the clap). In chronic infection, there may be gonococcemia which reveals (b) acral petechiae (Courtesy of R. Schift, MD, Rotterdam, the Netherlands) and (c) arthritis, characterized by erythema and swelling of the proximal interphalangeal joints (Courtesy of Michel Janier, MD, Paris, France).

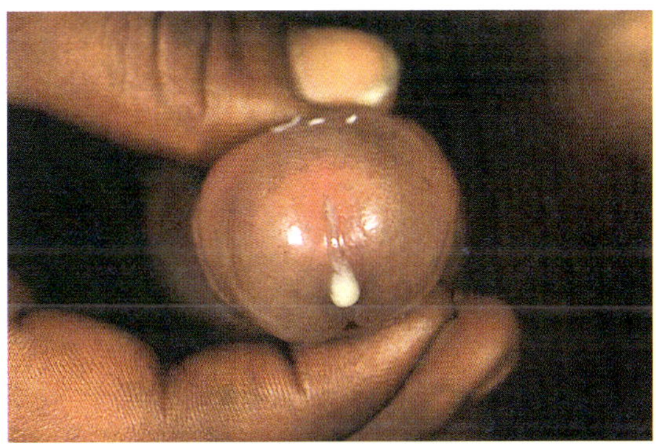

a

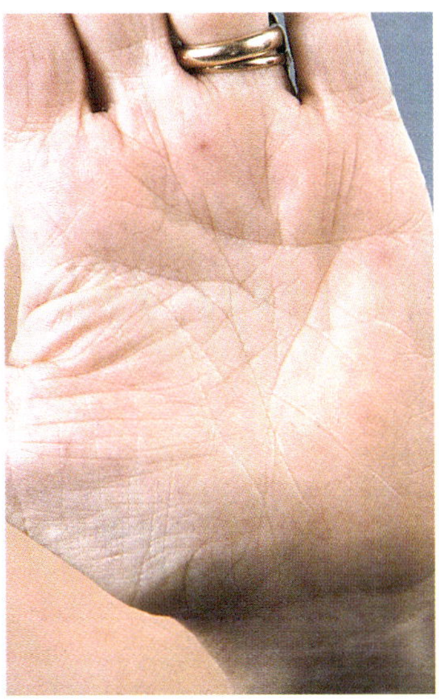

b

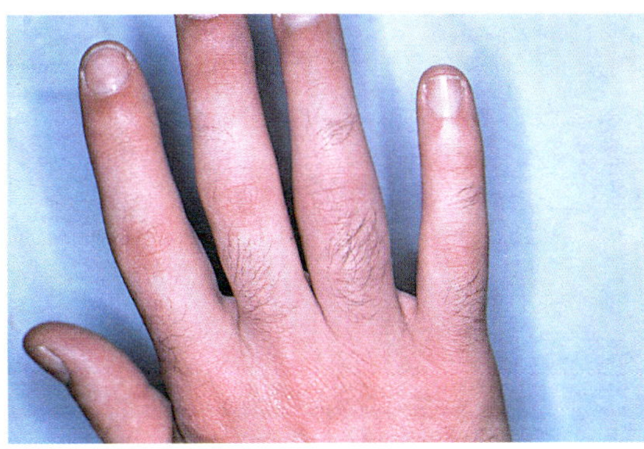

c

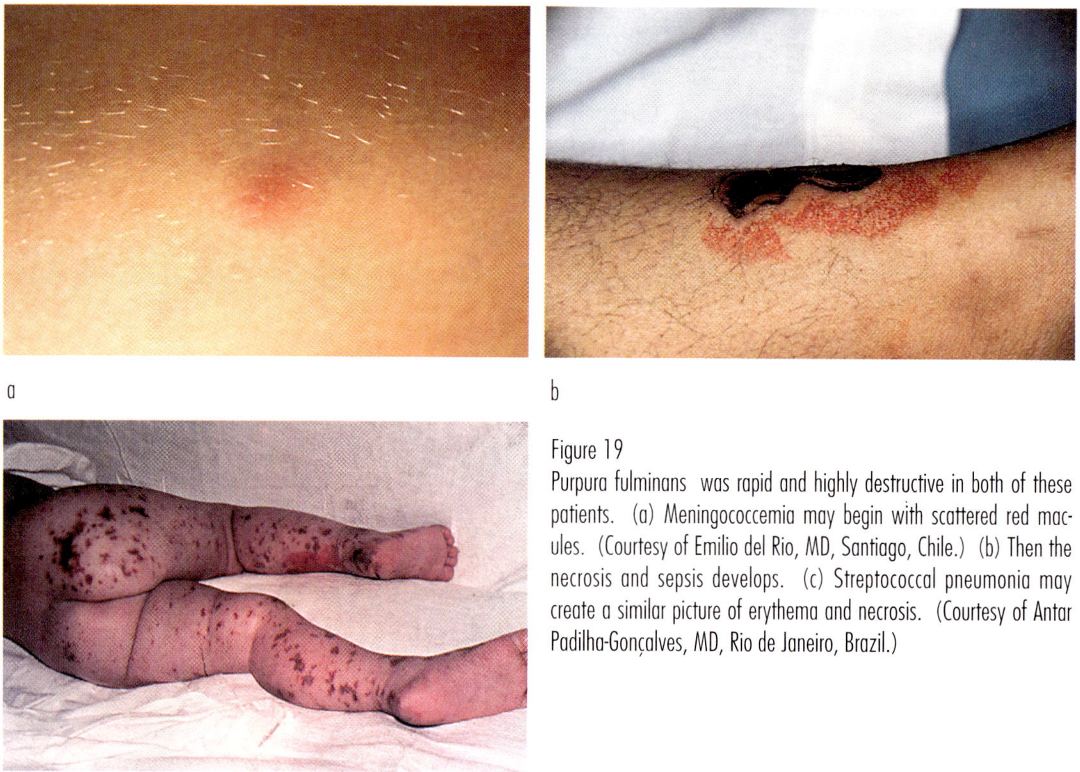

a

b

c

Figure 19
Purpura fulminans was rapid and highly destructive in both of these patients. (a) Meningococcemia may begin with scattered red macules. (Courtesy of Emilio del Rio, MD, Santiago, Chile.) (b) Then the necrosis and sepsis develops. (c) Streptococcal pneumonia may create a similar picture of erythema and necrosis. (Courtesy of Antar Padilha-Gonçalves, MD, Rio de Janeiro, Brazil.)

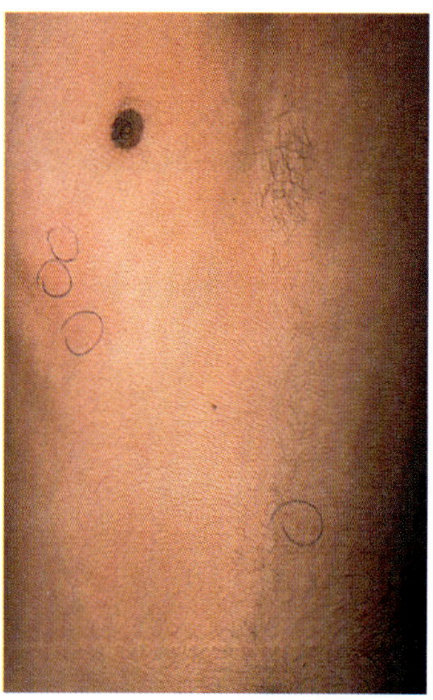

20

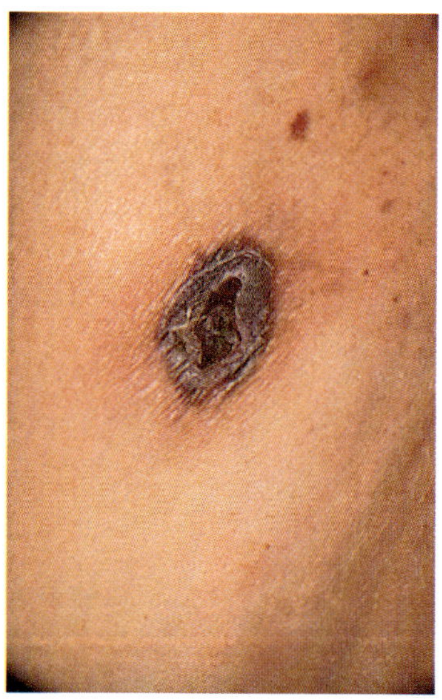

21

Figure 20
Salmonellosis may result in rose spots on the abdomen.

Figure 21
Ecthyma gangrenosum appears as an eschar with perilesional erythema. It may be confused with the eschar of the decubitus ulcer or with the necrosis due to heparin or coumarin therapy.

indurated, creating an ulcer covered by a central black eschar with surrounding erythema. The entire process can evolve within a few hours. Histologic examination shows a vasculitis involving both arteries and veins, while blood cultures will often grow the pathogen (Figure 21).

DIAGNOSIS

Cutaneous infections may range from demonstrating obvious signs and symptoms to being silent (Table 3). Usually, the redness, induration, and tenderness suggest a bacterial component. A smear that is gram stained may suggest an infection, and a bacterial culture may confirm this, but the diagnosis is made predominantly on the basis of clinical presentation, with laboratory confirmation being obtained as needed.

Table 3 Diagnostic Considerations

Clinical signs	Clinical symptoms	Laboratory findings	Microbiologic findings
redness	pruritus	leukocytosis	+ gram stain (white blood cells and stained bacterial components)
induration tenderness	polymorphonucleocytosis	elevated erythrocyte sedimentation rate	
headache	pain		+ culture
swelling	chills		
pustules	sweats		
purulent discharge	malaise		
serous discharge	headache		
scaling			
lymphangitis			
lymphadenopathy			
ulceration			

Adapted from Parish LC, Witkowski JA. Systemic management of cutaneous infections. Am J Med 1991;91(suppl 6A):106S-109S.

TREATMENT

Many cutaneous infections are diminished by compressing with Burow's solution 1:40 for 20 minutes tid. Saline or tap water compresses are also helpful. Superficial folliculitis and pyoderma respond to the use of topical antimicrobial agents, such as pseduomonic or fusidic acid ointment, applied bid to tid. Deeper and disseminated, more intense infections require systemic antimicrobials. The first choice, depending upon the offending organism, may be ampicillin–clavulanic acid bid, a cephalosporin, or a macrolide. Consideration may also be given to using a quinolone, particularly for gram-negative organisms (Table 4).

Table 4 Commonly Used Antimicrobial Agents

Agent	Amount	Time
penicillins		
penicillin v	250 mg qid	7–10 days
amoxicillin with clavulinc acid	500 mg tid	7–10days
dicloxacillin	250 mg qid	7–10 days
cephalosporins		
cefaclor	250 mg tid	7–10 days
cephalexin	250 mg qid	7–10 days
cefadroxil	1 gm qid	7–10 days
cefuroxime axetil	250 mg bid	7–10 days
cefprozil	500 mg qid	7–10days
cefpodoxime proxetil	400 mg bid	7–10 days
macrolides		
erythromycin	500 mg qid	7–10 days
clarithromycin	250 mg bid	7–10 days
azithromycin	500 mg qid	first day
	250 mg qid	next 4 days
tetracyclines		
tetracycline	500 mg qid	7–10 days
doxycycline	100 mg bid	first day
	50 mg bid	next 6–9 days
minocycline	200 mg initially	
	100 mg bid	next 7–10 days
quinolones		
ciprofloxacin	500 mg bid	7–10 days
ofloxacin	400 mg bid	7–10 days
topical		
neomycin ointment	tid	7–10 days
mupirocin ointment	tid	7–10 days

SUGGESTED READINGS

Aly R, Levit S. The changing spectrum of streptococcal and staphylococcal disease. Curr Opin Dermatol 1994;1:290–295.

Chartier C, Grosshans E. Erysipelas. Int J Dermatol 1990;29:459–467.

Craft JC. Antimicrobial Therapy. In: Parish LC, Millikan LE, Amer M, et al., eds. Global dermatology. New York:Springer-Verlag, 1994:311–316.

Demidovich CW, Wittler RR, Ruff ME. Impetigo: current etiology and comparison of penicillin, erythromycin, and cephalexin therapies. Am J Dis Child 1990;144:1313–1315.

Ducos M-H, Taieb A, Sarlangue J, et al. Cutaneous manifestations of Kawasaki disease. Ann Dermatol Venereol 1993;120:589–597.

Finch R. Skin and soft-tissue infections. Lancet 1988;ii:164–167.

Friter BS, Lucky AW. The perineal eruption of Kawasaki syndrome. Arch Dermatol 1988;124:1805–1810.

Haas AF. Antibiotic prophylaxis. Semin Dermatol 1994;13:27–34.

Johnson RA. Trends in dermatology: re-emergence of the infectious diseases. In: Sober AJ, Fitzpatrick TB, eds. Year book of dermatology 1991. St. Louis: Mosby–Year Book, 1991:xxi–xiv.

Leung DYM, Meissner HC, Fulton DR, et al. Toxic shock syndrome toxin-secreting Staphylococcus aureus in Kawasaki syndrome. Lancet 1993;342:1385–1387.

Lipsky BA. Diabetic foot infections: pathophysiology, diagnosis, and treatment. Int J Dermatol 1991;30:560–562.

Maibach HI, Aly R. Skin microbiology: relevance to clinical infection. New York: Springer-Verlag, 1981:1–354.

Mirensky Y, Parish LC, Witkowski JA. Recent advances in antimicrobial therapy of bacterial infection of the skin. Curr Opin Dermatol 1995;2:179–184.

Parish LC, Witkowski JA. Systemic management of cutaneous infections. Am J Med 1991;91(suppl 6A):106S–109S.

Parish LC, Witkowski JA. Cutaneous bacterial infections: how to manage primary, secondary, and tertiary lesions. Postgrad Med 1992;91:119–136.

Parish LC, Witkowski JA, Mirensky Y. Recent advances in antimicrobial therapy of bacterial infections of the skin. Curr Opin Dermatol 1994;1:263–270.

Roth RR, James WD. Microbiology of the skin: resident flora, ecology, infection. J Am Acad Dermatol 1989;20:367–390.

Sachs MK. Cutaneous cellulitis. Arch Dermatol 1991;127:493–496.

ADDITIONAL BACTERIAL INFECTIONS

Several bacteria in addition to staphylococci and streptococci cause cutaneous infections. Many of the diseases associated with these organisms have experienced a resurgence due to the rise in the number of immunocompromised patients and the increase in political and social upheavals.

Anthrax

Anthrax is known as the disease of the malignant pustule.

ETIOLOGY

This zoonosis is caused by *Bacillus anthracis*, an aerobic, spore-forming, large gram-positive rod containing two large plasmids $_{p}$X01 and $_{p}$X02. It is a destructive threat to sheep and goats and is often transmitted by contaminated wool, hairs, hides, or sheep carcasses. Periodic epidemics have occurred in the general population due to infected hairbrush bristles.

CLINICAL PRESENTATION

There are three forms of anthrax found in humans: (1) cutaneous, (2) pulmonary, and (3) gatrointestinal, which is less common. The cutaneous type can be divided into the dry and the edematous forms.

The dry form is relatively innocuous. It begins with a hemorrhagic area that quickly becomes a necrotic eschar (Figure 22a). The edematous form is characterized by initial fluid loss and subsequent vasoparalyisis leading to swelling. Both develop in areas of friction or trauma. This is exemplified by carpet weavers who held contaminated yarn with their lips or patients who used contaminated shave brushes to lather up their faces.

The malignant pustule or anthrax carbuncle, found near the onset of the disease, is actually an erythematous nodule that quickly evolves into a darker bluish red lesion with subcutaneous hemorrhage. The lesion is often pruritic (Figure 22b).

DIAGNOSIS

The diagnosis is made clinically, supported by gram staining of infected material. This shows gram-positive bacilli. Culture on nutrient agar or broth will reveal *B. anthracis*. An enzyme-linked immunosorbent assay (ELISA) for antibodies to the toxin, protective antigens, or lethal factor can also be used.

DIFFERENTIAL DIAGNOSIS

Anthrax may resemble urticaria, a carbuncle, or a furuncle in its early stages. The edematous type may be confused with bullous erysipelas or a second degree burn. A gram stain will distinguish this disease from other entities. When it is crusted, anthrax can mimic cowpox, a European orthopox virus infection.

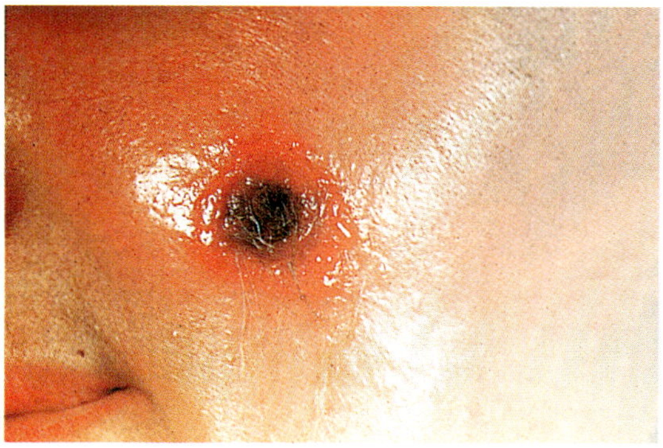

a

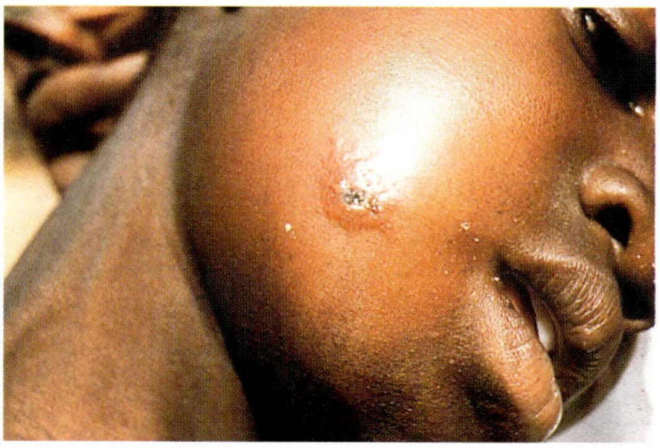

b

Figure 22
Anthrax often occurs on the face. It may appear (a) as a dry hemorrhagic crust (Courtesy of Margaret Gray Wood, MD, Philadelphia PA) or (b) as a malignant pustule, known also as the anthrax carbuncle, which is characterized by central ulceration and eschar formation, superimposed on an indurated plaque, and studded with vesicles (Courtesy of Wolfram Höffler, MD, Tübingen, Germany).

TREATMENT

Penicillin G, 600,000 units IV q12h for 5 days is the preferred treatment, although some penicillin resistance has been reported. Sulfadiazine, 3 gm and then 1 gm, q4h, erythromycin 250 mg q4h, or tetracycline 500 mg q4h are good alternative antimicrobial agents.

SUGGESTED READINGS

Brachman PS: Inhalation anthrax. Ann NY Acad Sci 1980;353:83–90.

Dutz W, Kohout-Dutz E. Anthrax. Int J Dermatol 1981;20:203–206.

Farrar WE. Anthrax: virulence and vaccines. Ann Int Med 1994;121:379–380.

Lewis-Jones MS, Baxby D, Cefai C, et al: Cowpox can mimic anthrax. Br J Dermatol 1993;129:625–627.

Cutaneous Diphtheria

Cutaneous diphtheria involves a variety of lesions from dermatitis to ulcers, but it is decidedly uncommon today in developed countries. Unfortunately, world turmoil has resulted in its resurgence in unexpected parts of the world.

ETIOLOGY

Corynebacterium diphtheriae is a gram-positive, pleomorphic rod that can invade skin traumatized by insect bites, irritation, or other infection. The bacteria are transmitted by respiratory spray or contact with infected skin, their pathogenicity being augmented by humidity and poor hygiene.

CLINICAL PRESENTATION

The lesions frequently present as punched-out ulcers (Figure 23a), although *C. diphtheriae* can cause pustules or eczematized dermatitis (Figure 23b). The ulcers appear as single defects or in multiple areas. Initially, they develop as pustules or vesicles, which over the ensuing days are transformed into a painful eschar or pseudoeschar. Within a week, the lesion becomes anesthetic with the eschar covering a hemorrhagic base.

DIAGNOSIS

The clinical picture is confirmed by bacteriologic culture and toxin production.

DIFFERENTIAL DIAGNOSIS

Because *C. diphtheriae* can create several different dermatologic pictures, the disease may also resemble a non-specific dermatitis.

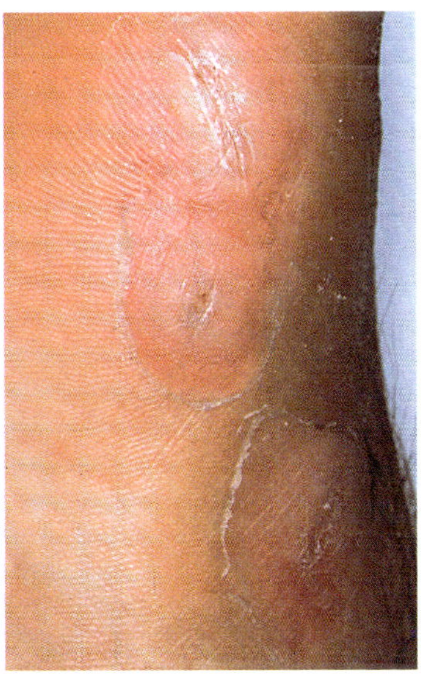

a

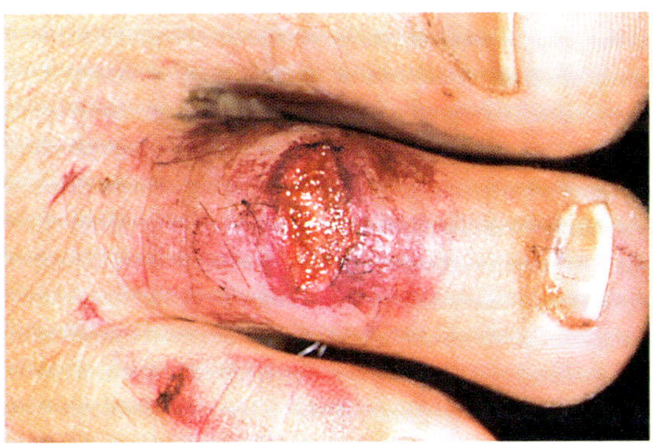

b

Figure 23
Cutaneous diphtheria may present itself as (a) punched-out ulcers with surrounding erythema, as shown on this ankle, or as (b) an eczematized area. (Courtesy of Wolfram Höffler, MD, Tübingen, Germany.)

TREATMENT

The toxin is eliminated by neutralization of the diphtheria antitoxin. The bacteria are reduced by the use of many agents ranging from penicillin G to tetracycline or erythromycin.

SUGGESTED READINGS

Cheb RT, Broome CV, Weinstein RA, et al. Diphtheria in the United States 1971–1981. Am J Public Health 1985;75:1393–1397.

Harnisch JP, Tronca E, Nolan CM, et al. Diphtheria among alcoholic urban adults. A decade of experience in Seattle. Ann Int Med 1989;111:71–82.

Hofler W. Cutaneous diphtheria. Int J Dermatol 1991;31:845–846.

ERYTHRASMA

Erythrasma is a superficial infection of the intertriginous areas.

ETIOLOGY

At one time thought to be a fungal infection, erythrasma is caused by *Corynebacterium minutussimum*, which may represent a group of aerobic corynebacteria that are a part of the normal skin flora. Growth of this diphtheroid on the skin is augmented by heat and humidity. Diabetes mellitus may also be a contributing factor.

CLINICAL PRESENTATION

Erythrasma appears as pink, scaling patches that later become brown, and are found in the axillae, inframammary area, crural region, and toe webs (Figures 24a,b). A generalized form can be seen on the trunk and upper aspects of the arms and legs, where the patches are well-defined and the scale lamellated. Mild itching may be present.

DIAGNOSIS

Examination under Wood's light shows a coral red fluorescence due to the coporphyrin III production of the bacteria. Unfortunately, bathing within 2 days of the examination may eliminate the color. Whereas KOH examination would be negative, a bacterial culture could reveal the gram-positive rods.

DIFFERENTIAL DIAGNOSIS

Dermatophytoses and candidosis may have similar clinical pictures but KOH scrapings and examination under Wood's lamp would confirm the appropriate diagnosis.

TREATMENT

Erythromycin, 250 mg qid for 5 days, is curative, as is tetracycline, 250 mg qid for 5 days. Erythromycin, fusidic acid, or antifungals applied topically can be equally helpful.

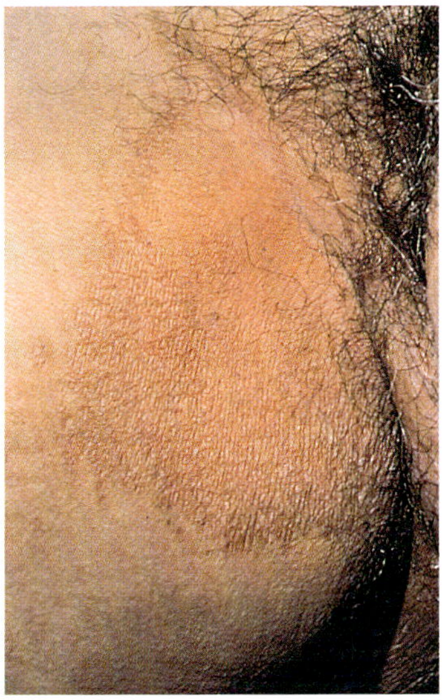

a

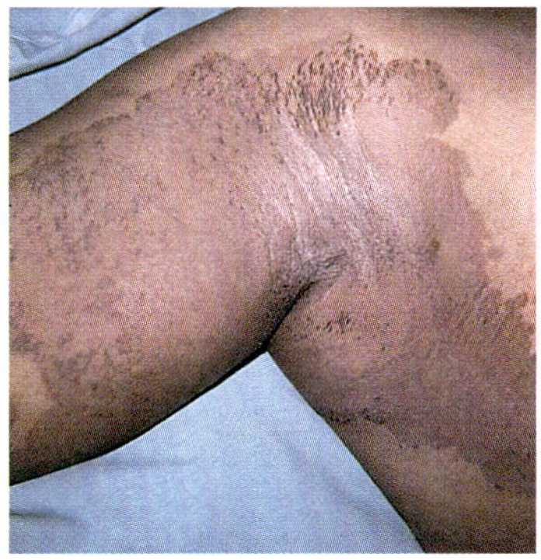

b

Figure 24
Erythrasma is characterized by (a) a tan scaling patch. Sometimes it can be more extensive, as seen in this patient's axilla (b).

SUGGESTED READINGS

Gollredge CL, Phillips G. Corynebacterium minutissimum infection. J Infect 1991;23:73–76.

Shelley WB, Shelley ED. Coexistent erythrasma, trichomycosis axillaris, and pitted keratolysis: An overlooked corynebacterial triad? J Am Acad Dermatol 1982;7:752–757.

Sindhuphak W, MacDonald E, Smith EB. Erythrasma: Overlooked or misdiagnosed? Int J Dermatol 1985;24:95–96.

TRICHOMYCOSIS AXILLARIS

Trichomycosis axillaris is a discoloration of the axillary hair.

ETIOLOGY

Corynebacterium tenuis, among other aerobic corynebacteria, is the causative agent and is gram-positive. It appears to proliferate only on axillary hairs and in the presence of moisture.

CLINICAL PRESENTATION

The hairs of the axillary vault become discolored and brittle. The color of the afflicted hairs are yellow, red, or black, indicating the synthesis of porphyrins by the bacteria. There is a rancid odor emanating from the adherent nodules. Infrequently, other body hairs may be involved, but the skin is not afflicted. Because there is hyperhidrosis associated with the condition, sweat carries the discoloration onto the adjacent clothing (Figure 25).

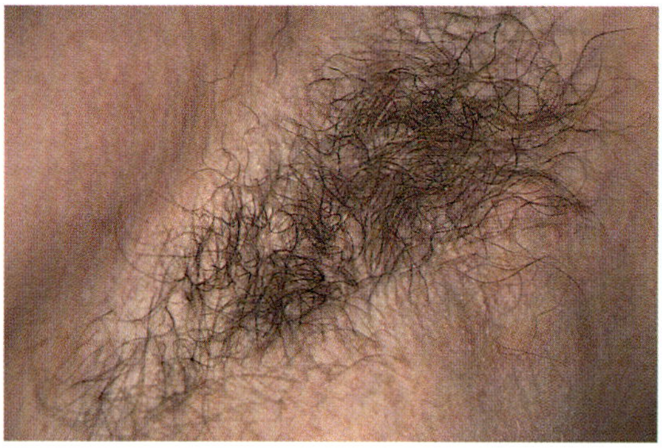

Figure 25
In trichomycosis axillaris there are yellowish concretions on the hair shafts.

DIAGNOSIS

The clinical picture may be confirmed by using Wood's light which will fluoresce the afflicted areas. KOH examination of the hairs will show short bacillary forms. Bacterial culture will reveal the organism.

DIFFERENTIAL DIAGNOSIS

The staining of the clothing may be confused with chromhidrosis, and the hair may initially be thought to have louse nits. Black piedra may also be considered.

TREATMENT

Cutting the hair and washing regularly with antibacterial soaps will eliminate the disease.

SUGGESTED READINGS

Freeman RG, McBride M, Knox JM. Pathogenesis of trichomycosis axillaris. Arch Dermatol 1969;100:90–95.

Shelley WB, Miller MA. Electron microscopy, histochemistry, and microbiology of bacterial adhesion in trichomycosis axillaris. J Am Acad Dermatol 1984;10:1005–1014.

Shelley WB, Shelley ED. Coexistent erythrasma, trichomycosis axillaris, and pitted keratolysis: an overlooked corynebacterial triad? J Am Acad Dermatol 1982;7:752–757.

Pitted Keratolysis

Pitted keratolysis is a superficial erosive disease of the soles.

ETIOLOGY

Moisture and occlusive shoes create the environment for the causative gram-positive filamentous organism to proliferate. The bacillus appears to be a corynbacterium; however, *Dermatophilus congolenis*, an actinomycete, and *Micrococcus sedentarius* have been recovered experimentally. Possibly, more than one organism may be involved.

CLINICAL PRESENTATION

The sole and toes show pitted lesions that may coalesce to form larger depressions. The pits range from skin color to brown. The surrounding skin is often white and macerated due to hyperhidrosis. A typical fetid odor is present. The initial itching or burning progresses into pain as the patient tries to walk or stand for more than a few minutes (Figure 26).

DIAGNOSIS

The clinical picture is confirmed by finding gram-positive coccobacilli in the stratum corneum. The organism cannot be readily cultured.

DIFFERENTIAL DIAGNOSIS

Extensive tinea pedis, mosaic warts, basal cell nevus syndrome, and even Darier's disease could be considered, but the negative KOH scraping, the positive gram stain, and lack of lesions elsewhere on the body would distinguish these diseases from pitted keratosis.

TREATMENT

Washing with soap on a daily basis will prevent the condition. Initially, soaking in Burow's 1:40 solution for 10 minutes tid followed by applications of antibiotic acne lotions such as erythromycin or clindamycin will eliminate the condition. Aluminum chlorhexahydrate applications are also helpful in reducing the predisposing hyperhidrosis.

SUGGESTED READINGS

Nordstrom KM, McGinley KJ, Cappiello L, et al. Pitted keratolysis: the role of Micrococcus sedentarius. Arch Dermatol 1987;123:1320–1325.

Shelley WB, Shelley ED: Coexistent erythrasma, trichomycosis axillaris, and pitted keratolysis: an overlooked corynebacterial triad? J Am Acad Dermatol 1982;7:752–757.

Zaias N. Pitted and ringed keratolysis. A review and update. J Am Acad Dermatol 1982;7:787–791.

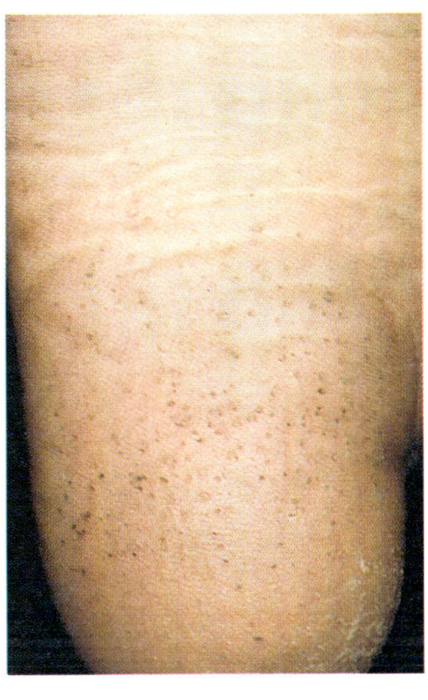

Figure 26
Pitted keratolysis is characterized by discrete punched-out defects in the stratum corneum.

Erysipeloid

Erysipeloid is a zoonotic infection often found in fishery and abattoir workers. It has been known as *erysipeloid of Rosenbach, fish handler's disease, crab dermatitis,* and *blubber finger.*

ETIOLOGY

Erysipelothrix rhusiopathiae is a gram-positive bacillus that is a facultative aerobe and is related to *Listeria monocytogenes*. It causes erysipeloid in humans and swine erysipelas in pigs. The bacterium is found in pigs, turkeys, crabs, and saltwater fish. Infections usually occur during the warm months and are spread by contact with the animal or fish as well as their by-products.

CLINICAL PRESENTATION

Three types of erysipeloid are recognized. In the *localized cutaneous form*, the characteristic raised, tender, purplish lesion appears between two days and a week following injury. There may be associated lymphadenopathy, malaise, and localized burning and pain. The lesion, which is frequently found on the hand, resolves within a few weeks (Figure 27). The *diffuse cutaneous form* has similar morphology; however, there are multiple lesions on various parts of the body. Instead of dissipating within a week, the condition may last a month or more, sometimes with relapses occurring up to four years later.

The *systemic form* resembles the localized form, but there may be generalized malaise, endocarditis, pleural effusions, and septic arthritis. Septicemia has even occurred. This form can smolder for many weeks without therapy.

DIAGNOSIS

In addition to the morphology, the diagnosis is suggested by a positive gram stain and confirmed by isolating the pathologic organism on culture. Unfortunately, these techniques are infrequently successful.

DIFFERENTIAL DIAGNOSIS

Cellulitis or erysipelas may be confused with erysipeloid. Gram stains and bacterial cultures may be helpful in establishing the correct diagnosis.

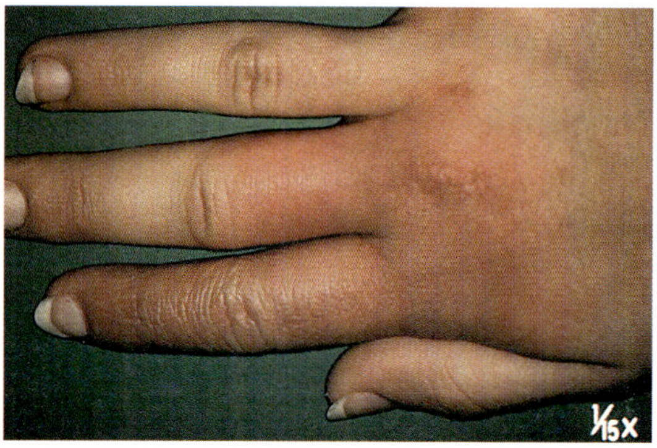

Figure 27
Erysipeloid may be recognized by the tender purplish induration on the fingers. (Courtesy of Guy Chabeau, MD, Lyon, France.)

TREATMENT

The most expedient treatment is the rapid initiation of therapy using penicillin, 2 to 3 million units daily, given in divided doses. Alternative measures include cephalosporins or macrolides. Sulfonamides have also been used.

SUGGESTED READINGS

Barnett JH, Estes SA, Winman JA, et al. Erysipeloid. J Am Acad Dermatol 1983;9:116–123.

Klauder JV, Righter LL, Harkins MJ. A distinctive and severe form of erysipeloid among fish handlers. Arch Dermatol Syphilol 1926; 14: 662–678.

Molin G, Soderlind O, Ursing J, et al. Occurrence of Erysipelothrix rhusiopathiae on pork and in pig slurry, and the distribution of specific antibodies in abattoir workers. J Appl Bacteriol 1989;67:347–352.

Reboli AC, Farrar WE. Erysipelothrix rhusiopathiae: an occupational pathogen. Clin Microbiol Rev 1989; 2:354–359.

LISTERIOSIS

Listeriosis is a multisystemic infection found most commonly in pregnant women, their fetuses, and immunocompromised patients.

ETIOLOGY

Listeria monocytogenes is a gram-positive rod that is a facultative anaerobe and causes intracellular infection. Although rare, seven other strains of *Listeria* are pathogenic and these bacilli are related to the *Erysipelothrix* bacillus. The organism is found in contaminated food, particularly dairy products. It causes circling disease or basilar meningoencephalitis in cattle and sheep.

CLINICAL PRESENTATION

The cutaneous findings are highly variable depending on the condition of the patient. In infants, there are petechiae and pustules or red papules on the body. The lesions are widespread and many appear as microabscesses (i.e., granulomatosis infantisepticum) (Figure 28).

Patients who have contracted the disease by handling animals develop papules and pustules at the site of contact. Within a few days, axillary lymphadenopathy, fever, and malaise develop. A third constellation of signs occurs in the oculoglandular type, with the development of preauricular lymphadenitis and acute conjunctivitis.

In many patients, particularly those with depressed immunity from steroid administration or with concomitant diseases, there is fulminant septicemia, meningitis, pneumonitis, urethritis, and malaise that is reminiscent of infectious mononucleosis. Without treatment, the prognosis is poor.

DIAGNOSIS

Culture obtained from the skin, blood, or spinal fluid may grow the bacillus, which can mimic a diphtheroid. A skin biopsy may reveal focal necrosis and perivascular infiltrates.

DIFFERENTIAL DIAGNOSIS

Toxoplasmosis, rubella, and disseminated herpetic infections may give a similar appearance in infants. Pyogenic infections should be considered in adults, as should such rickettsial diseases as Rocky Mountain spotted fever.

TREATMENT

Ampicillin is the antibacterial agent of choice. Penicillin is highly effective. In the penicillin-allergic patient, trimethoprim-sulfamethoxazole, erythromycin, or tetracycline may be used.

SUGGESTED READINGS

Cain DB, McCann VL. An unusual case of cutaneous listeriosis. J Clin Microbiol 1986;23:976–977.

Farber JM, Peterkin PI. Listeria monocytogenes, a food-borne disease. Microbiol Rev 1991;55:476–511.

Riviera L, Dubini F, Bellotti MG. Listeria monocytogenes infections: the organism, its pathogenicity and antimicrobial drug susceptibility. Microbiologica 1993;16:189–203.

Schlech WF III. Listeriosis: epidemiology, virulence and the significance of contaminated foddstuffs. J Hosp Infect 1991;19:211–224.

Schlech A, Swaminathan B, Broome CV. Epidemiology of human listeriosis. Clin Microbiol Rev 1991;4:169–183.

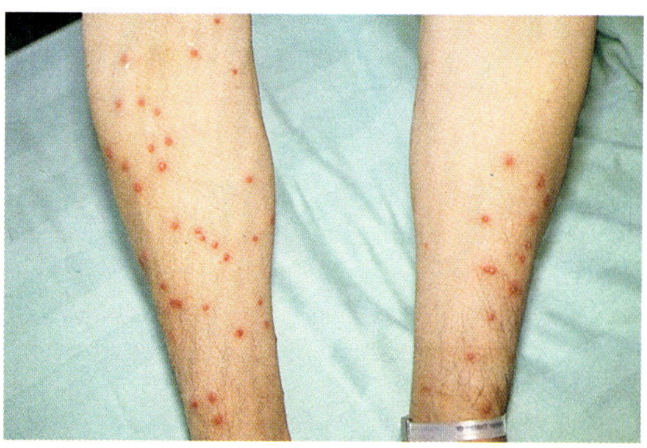

Figure 28
Listerosis is presented as discrete erythematous papules on the legs. (Courtesy of David B. Cain, Medicine Hat, ALB, Canada.)

Tularemia

Tularemia, also known as *deerfly* or *rabbit fever*, is a multifaceted granulomatous disease.

ETIOLOGY

Francisella (Pasturella) tularensis is a small gram-negative bacillus that may have coccoid forms and has a strong endotoxin. The bacterium is found in rabbits, rodents, birds, and reptiles. It is accidentally spread to humans by arthropod bites, contact, contaminated food, or even inhalation. Ticks, such as *Dermacentor variabilis, D. endersoni*, and *Amblyomma americanum*, appear to be the most significant vector, but deerflies, fleas, lice, and mosquitoes have also been implicated in the spread of the disease. *F. tularensis* creates an intracellular infection in the reticuloendothelial system.

CLINICAL PRESENTATION

One to nine days following inoculation, there is a rapid onset of fever, chills, malaise, and arthralgia. There are six types of tularemia: ulceroglandular, oculoglandular, glandular, oropharyngeal, pneumonic, and typhoidal. Cutaneous manifestations include macules, papules, pustules, and vesicles, giving a picture of toxic erythema, sometimes accompanied by erythema nodosum. Frequently, the redness is more prominent on the arms and upper aspects of the trunk.

The inoculation site is usually found on the hand or the exposed part of the arm, if transmitted by a flying organism, or the armpit, groin, or beltline, if transmitted by a crawling organism. In the ulceroglandular type, the small purplish, painful nodule, which appears shortly after the constitutional signs, deteriorates into a punched-out ulcer within a few days (Figure 29a). The lesion may by single or multiple. In the glandular type, lymphadenopathy, lymphangitis, and even buboes occur (Figure 29b).

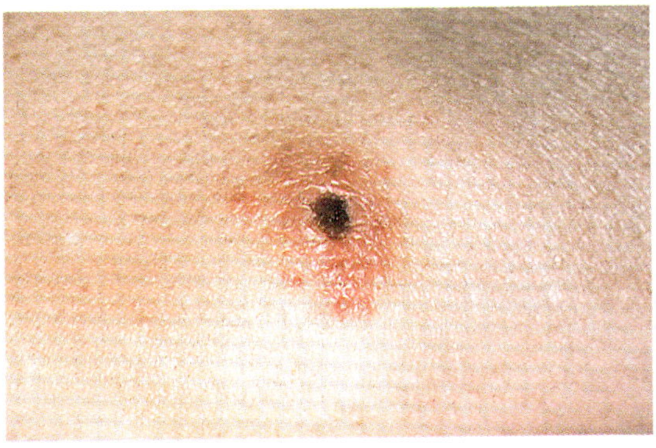

a

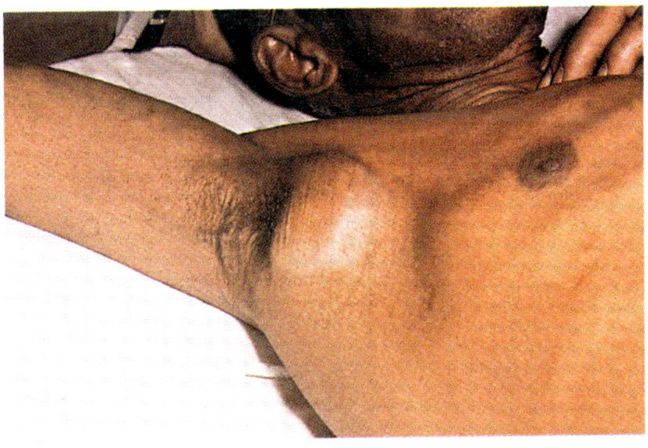

b

Figure 29
(a) Tularemia begins as a central eschar surrounded by erythema. Later it becomes crusted. (b) The markedly enlarged axillary lymph nodes were the only cutaneous findings. (Courtesy of Peyton Weary, MD, Charlotteville, VA.)

SUGGESTED READINGS

Açay MC, Oral ET, Yenigün M, et al. Pasteurella multocida ulceration on the penis. Int J Dermatol 1993;32:519–520.

Brue C, Chosidow O. Pasteurella multocida wound infection and cellulitis. Int J Dermatol 1994;33:471–473.

Brue C, Chosidow O, Gueorguieva E, et al. Cellulitis graves a Pasteurella multocida; deux observations. Ann Dermatol Venereol 1992;119:859–860.

Goldstein EJC, Reinhardt JF, Murray PM, et al. Outpatient therapy of bite wounds: demographic data, bacteriology, and a prospective, randomized trial of amoxicillin/clavulanic acid versus penicillin±dicloxacillin. Int J Dermatol 1987;26:123–127.

Kumar A, Devlin HR, Vellend H. Pasteurella multocida meningitis in an adult: case report and review. Rev Infect Dis 1990;12:440–448.

Swartz MN, Kunz LJ. Pasteurella multocida infection in man: report of two cases — meningitis and infected cat bite. N Engl J Med 1959;261:889–893.

Tindall JP, Harrison CM. Pasteurella multocida infections following animal injuries, especially cat bites. Arch Dermatol 1972;105:412–416.

BOTRYOMYCOSIS

Botryomycosis is a rare form of mycetoma which is characterized by microscopic granules and generally is treatable.

ETIOLOGY

Staphylococcus aureus is the most common organism implicated, but gram-negative organisms, including *Pseudomonas aeruginosa* and Proteus species have been recovered from some patients. The disease appears to develop following trauma and represents a compromise between the virulence of the pathogen and the resistence of the host.

CLINICAL PRESENTATION

There are two types of botryomycosis: (1) the visceral form, usually found in the lungs and less commonly in the tongue, kidney, prostate, and liver, and (2) a cutaneous form that can appear anywhere on the body. The latter begins as an inflammatory nodule that enlarges into draining sinuses with ulcerations and fistulae. The lesion may then extend into the subcutaneous tissue and bone (Figure 31a,b). White or yellow grains are seen.

DIAGNOSIS

Biopsy of the lesion will reveal grapelike granules and bacteria, surrounded by necrosis and pus. The eosinophilic matrix (Splendore-Hoeppli phenomenon) represents the antibody-antigen compromise.

DIFFERENTIAL DIAGNOSIS

Initially, prurigo nodularis or a foreign body may be confused with botryomycosis. In later stages of the disease, mycetomas and actinomycosis need to be distinguished by culture and histopathologic examination.

TREATMENT

Antimicrobial therapy with a penicillin, cephalosporin, or quinolone is effective, although surgical excision may be needed.

SUGGESTED READINGS

Bishop GF, Greer KE, Horwitz DA. Pseudomonas botryomycosis. Arch Dermatol 1976;112:1568–1570.

Brunken RC, Lichon-Chao N, van den Broek H. Immunologic abnormalities in botryomycosis. J Am Acad Dermatol 1983;9:428–434.

Findlay GH, Vismer HF. Botryomycosis: some African cases. Int J Dermatol 1990;29:340–344.

Hacker P. Botryomycosis. Int J Dermatol 1983;22:455–458.

Patterson JW, Kitces EN, Neafie RC. Cutaneous botryomycosis in a patient with acquired immunodeficiency syndrome. J Am Acad Dermatol 1987;16:238–242.

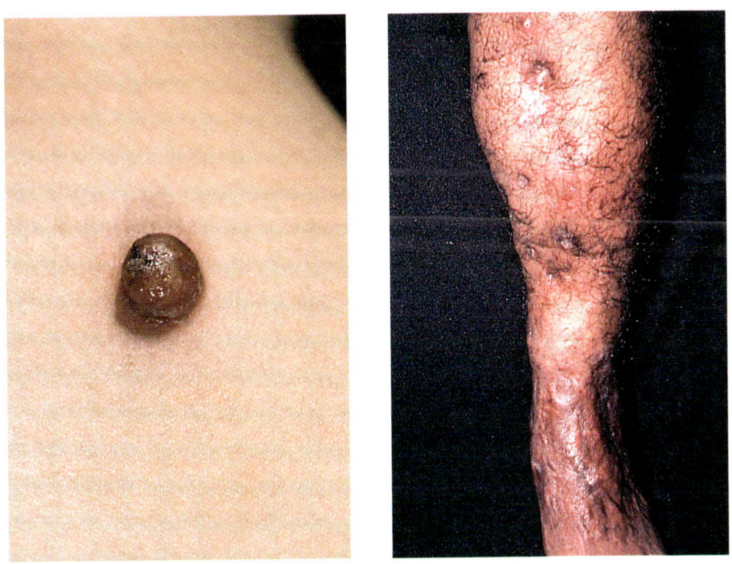

a b

Figure 31
(a) Botryomycosis appears as a purplish nodule with almost no surrounding swelling. (Courtesy of Stephania Jablonska, MD, Warsaw, Poland.) (b) It also can present as multiple erythematous to purplish nodules. (Courtesy of Roberto Arenas, MD, Mexico City, Mexico.)

Rhinoscleroma

Rhinoscleroma is an invasive granulomatous disease found on the nose, from where it invades the upper respiratory tract and leads to sclerosis.

ETIOLOGY

Klebsiella rhinoscleromatis is a short, gram-negative organism that enters the nasal mucosa and the upper respiratory tract.

CLINICAL PRESENTATION

The disease begins as a common cold with headache and a runny nose. The nasal discharge becomes foul smelling, with the mucosal surfaces being crusted and friable. This is followed by infiltration of the nose and later the pharynx and larynx, accompanied by redness, necrosis, and drainage (Figure 32). Finally, there is nodular destruction so that the nose and upper lip are deformed. This results in compromised breathing.

DIAGNOSIS

Finding the pathogen in the culture of the tissue confirms the diagnosis. Histopathologically, there is an inflammatory process with Russell bodies and plasma cells. Mikulicz's cells resemble large, swollen histiocytes containing bacilli.

DIFFERENTIAL DIAGNOSIS

Granulomatous deep fungal diseases, such as paeacoccidioidomycosis and North American blastomycosis, may be considered. Leishmaniasis may create a similar clinical picture.

TREATMENT

Antimicrobial therapy with quinolones, cephalosporins, trimethoprim-sulfamethoxazole, rifampin, or chloramphenicol in therapeutic doses is very useful in the early stage. Treatment should be continued for at least 6 months. When stenosis has occurred, cold steel or laser surgery may be indicated.

SUGGESTED READINGS

Batsakis JG, el-Naggar AK. Rhinoscleroma and rhinosporidiosis. Ann Otol Rhinol Laryngol 1992;101:879–892.

Convit J, Kerdel-Vegas F, Gordon B. Rhinoscleroma: review and presentation of a case. Arch Dermatol 1961;84:55–62.

Kerdel-Vegas F, Convit J, Gordon B, et al. Rhinoscleroma. Springfield, IL: Charles C Thomas, 1963.

Sosa R, Garcia E, Alanos A. Rhinoscleroma. Dermatol Rev Mex 1994;38:199–201.

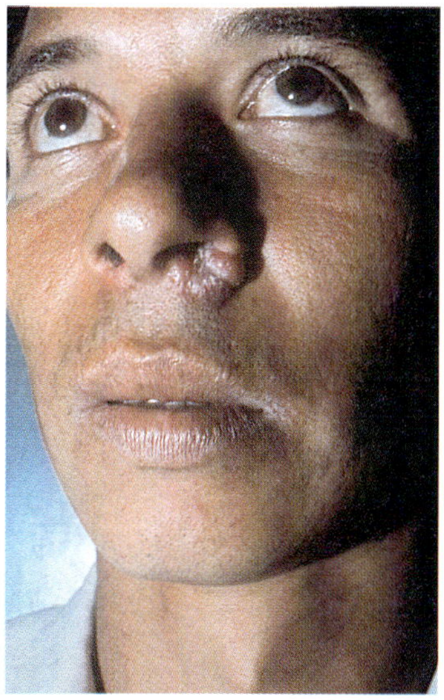

Figure 32
Rhinoscleroma was diagnosed early in this Brazilian man, when the physician recognized the characteristic red, crusted hypertrophic papules. (Courtesy of Sebastião AP Sampãio, MD, São Paulo, Brazil.)

Necrotizing Fasciitis

Necrotizing fasciitis, also called *necrotizing erysipelas* or *hospital gangrene*, is a generalized term for a destructive process leading to gangrene (Figure 33a). A specific type of necrotizing fasciitis is Fournier's gangrene, a rare necrotizing process involving the male genitalia and the surrounding tissue, sometimes extending to the buttocks (Figure 33b).

ETIOLOGY

ß-hemolytic Streptococci, Group A, as well as other organisms, act sinergistically to create a rapidly destructive process. Some bacteria directly create the necrosis, where as others participate through exotoxins or endotoxins. There is usually preceding trauma.

CLINICAL PRESENTATION

The disease represents the rapid development of gangrene. Although the onset may be sudden, there can be a smoldering onset with itching, pain, and malaise, followed by erythema and swelling of the tissues. Gangrene then ensues.

Necrotizing fasciitis can involve any part of the body, but Fournier's gangrene, by definition, is limited to the scrotum, penis, and perineum. An odiferous slough is created that may expose the testicles or other underlying tissue. Patients often have poor hygiene, and there is a history of trauma or recent surgery.

DIAGNOSIS

A positive bacterial culture will support the clinical diagnosis.

DIFFERENTIAL DIAGNOSIS

Necrosis of the skin can be caused by a wide variety of infectious chemical or physical agents as well as by ischemia. Finding a pathogen in the tissue would suggest necrotizing fasciitis.

TREATMENT

Antimicrobial therapy, using quinolones or cephalosporins, is recommended. Because the disease is rapidly destructive and, in the case of Fournier's gangrene, aggressive therapy in up to 20% of the cases is recommended. Surgical debridement and reconstruction are usually needed.

SUGGESTED READINGS

Chelsom J, Halstenson, Huga T, et al. Necrotizing fasciitis due to Group A Streptococci in western Norway: incidence and clinical features. Lancet 1994;344:1111–1115.

Feingold DS. Gangrenous and crepitant cellulitis. J Am Acad Dermatol 1982;6:289(299.

Giulliano A, Lewis F Jr, Hadley K, et al. Bacteriology of necrotizing fasciitis. Am J Surg 1977;134:52–57.

Jackson R, Bell M. Phagedena: gangrenous and necrotic ulcerations of skin and subcutaneous tissue. Can Med Assoc J 1982;126:363–368.

Loudon I. Necrotizing fasciitis, hospital gangrene, and phagedena. Lancet 1994;334:1416–1419.

Quintal D, Jackson R. Necrosis of the skin. In: Moschella SL, Hurley HJ, eds. Dermatology. Philadelphia: WB Saunders, 1993:1206–1214.

Scott SD, Dawes RFH, Tate JJT, et al. The practical management of Fournier's gangrene. Ann R Coll Surg Engl 1988;70:16–20.

Singh S, Lynfield YL, Gruber H. Fournier's gangrene of the scrotum. Int J Dermatol 1975;14:508–509.

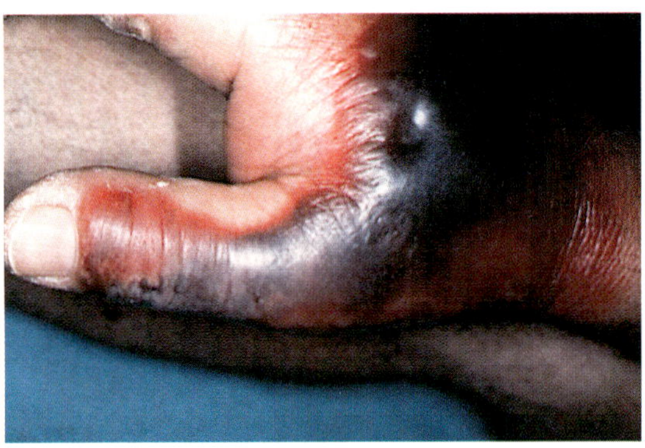

a

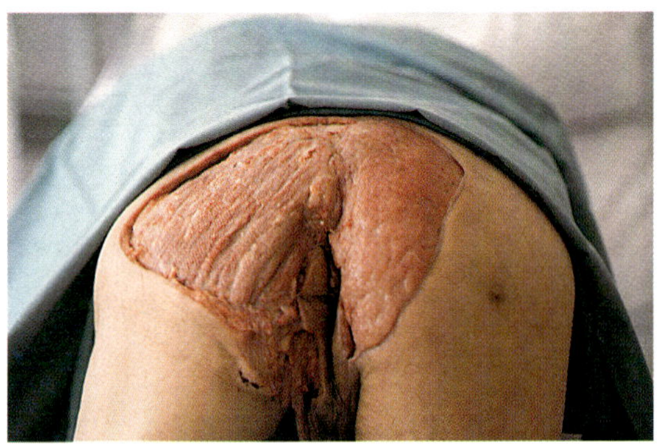

b

Figure 33
(a) Necrotizing fasciitis appeared as a purplish edematous process on the patientís hand. (Courtesy of Selim Aractingi, MD, Paris, France.) (b) Fournier's gangrene resulted in marked destruction to this patient's buttocks. (Courtesy of Alberto Bordallo Cortina, MD, Javea, Spain.)

Vibrio Infection

Vibrio infection has become an increasingly recognized necrotizing disease associated with exposure to shellfish.

ETIOLOGY

Vibrio vulnificus is a gram-negative bacillus that is facultatively anaerobic and is found in seawater, fish, and shellfish. Patients with decreased immunity due to viral infections and with hepatic dysfunction, particularly from alcoholism, and diabetes mellitus are prone to this destructive infection. Healthy people who are fish handlers may also contract infection from these bacteria.

CLINICAL PRESENTATION

The destructive process develops either in abrasions in patients exposed to raw shellfish or contaminated seawater or in patients ingesting raw seafood. Between 12 and 72 hours after exposure to the bacteria, chills, fever, nausea, and vomiting may begin, accompanied by the appearance of red to purple macules and patches on the back in most of the patients. The skin lesions progress into vesicles, bullae, pustules, and necrosis leading to ulcerations (Figure 34). The patient may also have necrotizing fasciitis and osteomyelitis. An ominous sign is hypotension early in the course of the disease. Disease occuring from contact appears on the hands or legs.

DIAGNOSIS

Obtaining a positive culture for *V. vulnificus* will confirm the diagnosis.

DIFFERENTIAL DIAGNOSIS

This infection may appear to be due to a variety of destructive bacteria. Necrotizing vasculitis may also be considered.

TREATMENT

Antimicrobial therapy (i.e., quinolones, cephalosporins, and tetracyclines) should be instituted immediately, as *V. vulnificus* infections are rapidly progressive, leading to septic shock and even death. Necrotic tissue should be debrided as quickly as possible.

SUGGESTED READINGS

Howard RJ, Bennett NT. Infections caused by halophilic marine Vibrio bacteria. Ann Surg 1993;217:525–530.

Koenig KL, Mueller J, Rose T. Vibrio vulnificus. Hazards on the half shell. West Med J 1991;155:421–422.

Park SD, Shon HS, Joh NJ. Vibrio vulnificus septicemia in Korea: clinical and epidemiologic findings in seventy patients. J Am Acad Dermatol 1991;24:397–403.

Tyring SK, Lee PC. Hemorrhagic bullae associated with Vibrio vulnificus septicemia. Arch Dermatol 1986;122:818–820.

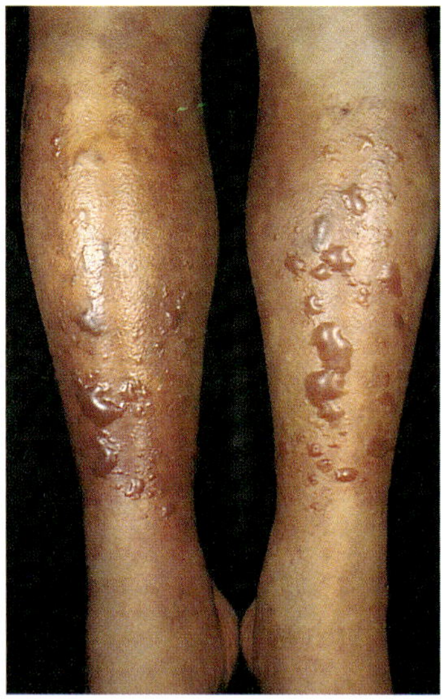

Figure 34
Vibrio infection occurred in this 55-year-old man after he ate contaminated oysters. Within several hours, purplish bullae had appeared. (Courtesy of Seok Don Park, MD, Iri City, Korea.)

Chancroid

Chancroid, sometimes known as the soft chancre, is a sexually transmitted disease that is now found worldwide.

ETIOLOGY

The causative agent is *Haemophilus ducreyi* (*Ducrey's bacillus*), a gram-negative, bipolar staining rod that creates ulcerations a week after exposure.

CLINICAL PRESENTATION

The initial lesion is a tender papule that develops within 24 hours of exposure. During the next several days, it becomes irregular, ulcerated, and painful. The soft chancre has a sharp border, but there may be undermining of this shallow ulceration with necrosis and friable tissue. Although there may be a single ulcer, multiple lesions are common due to autoinoculation (Figure 35). A week later, inguinal lymphadenopathy may be found. The lesions may become fluctuant and ulcerate. The ulcers are usually located on the genitalia at sites subject to trauma. A *bubo* is an enlarged, tender, inflammed lymphnode; it does not need to ulcerate.

DIAGNOSIS

A gram stain will show gram-negative rods. Cultures are successful in only 30% of cases, even with Mueller-Hinton agar or gonococcal agar base with chloramphenicol.

DIFFERENTIAL DIAGNOSIS

Primary syphilis differs by having a chancre without necrotic tissue. Herpes progenital-is may be confirmed by a Tzank smear.

TREATMENT

Several antimicrobial agents can be used successfully: erythromycin, 500 mg qid for 7 days; ceftriaxone, 250 mg IM; or ciprofloxacin, 500 mg bid for 3 days.

SUGGESTED READINGS

Goens JL, Schwartz RA, De Wolf K. Mucocutaneous manifestations of selected sexually transmitted diseases: chancroid, lymphogranuloma venereum, and granuloma inguinale. Am Fam Physician 1994;49:423–425.

Jones CC, Rosen T. Cultural diagnosis of chancroid. Arch Dermatol 1991;127:1823 –1827.

Neumann RA, Knobler RM, Aberer E, et al. Incidence of chancroid in Vienna from 1980 to 1988. Int J Dermatol 1989;28:393–396.

Parish LC, Seghal VN, Buntin DM. Color atlas of sexually transmitted diseases. New York: Igaku-Shoin, 1991:37–45.

Ronald AR. Chancroid. In Parish LC, Gschnait F, eds. Sexually transmitted diseases: a guide for clinicians. New York: Springer-Verlag, 1989:78–89.

Van Dyck E, Piot P. Laboratory techniques in the investigation of chancroid, lymphogranuloma venereum and donovanosis. Genitourin Med 1992;68:130–133.

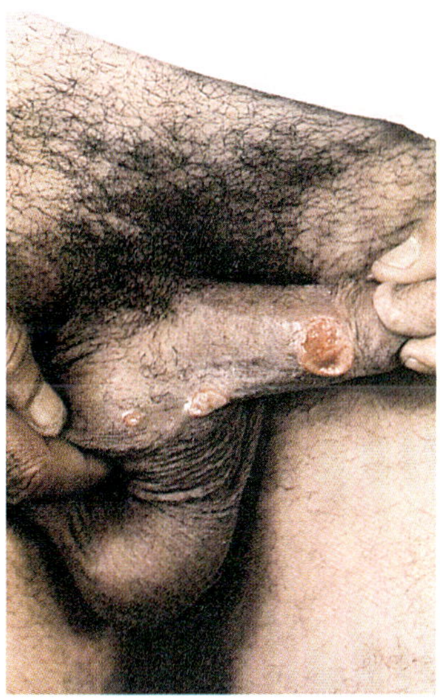

Figure 35
Chancroid may have several chancres. These lesions are characterized by sharp borders, superficial ulcerations, and dirty bases.

Granuloma Inguinale

Granuloma inguinale, also known as *donovanosis*, is a so-called minor venereal disease that is found in the United States and elsewhere, on occasion.

ETIOLOGY

Calymmatobacterium granulomatis is a gram-negative bacterium. Although it resembles the Klebsiella species, it has not been grown reliably. There is evidence that it may be a protozoan.

CLINICAL PRESENTATION

Within 3 to 90 days following sexual exposure, a papule appears. This gradually erodes and remains clean without pus. Four types are known: ulcerative, hypertrophic, necrotic, and sclerotic. The inguinal area may swell, being called a *pseudobubo*, and even ulcerate, although lymphadenopathy does not occur (Figure 36).

DIAGNOSIS

Smears of the lesions show Donovan bodies that appear in the cytoplasm of mononuclear cells stained with Giemsa. The organism has not been grown routinely. Histopathologic confirmation is obtained when a massive mononuclear cell infiltrate and Donovan bodies with plasma cells are found in the dermis.

DIFFERENTIAL DIAGNOSIS

Other sexually transmitted diseases may present with a similar genital ulcer.

TREATMENT

Sulfamethoxazole (400 mg) and trimethoprim (80 mg) bid for 2 weeks is recommended. Tetracycline, 500 mg qid or erythromycin, 500 mg qid for the same time period is satisfactory, but may fail.

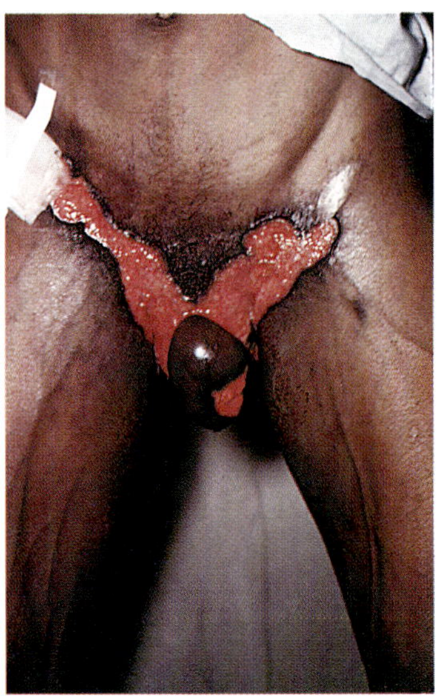

Figure 36
Granuloma inguinale involves ulcerations extending along the inguinal crease. (Courtesy of Bertram Shaffer, MD, Collection of the College of Physicians of Philadelphia.)

SUGGESTED READINGS

Niemel PL, Engelkens HJ, van der Meijden W, et al. Donovanosis (granuloma inguinale) still exists. Int J Dermatol 1992;31:244–246.

Parish LC, Sehgal VN, Buntin DM. Color atlas of sexually transmitted diseases. New York: Igaku-Shoin, 1991:95–102.

Sehgal VN. Granuloma inguinale. In Parish LC, Gschnait F, eds. Sexually transmitted diseases: a guide for clinicians. New York: Springer-Verlag, 1989:105–120.

Sehgal VN, Prasad ALS. Donovanosis: current clinical concepts. Int J Dermatol 1986;25:8–16.

Sehgal VN, Sharma HK. Donovanosis. J Dermatol 1992;19:932–946.

Van Dyck E, Piot P. Laboratory techniques in the investigation of chancroid, lymphogranuloma venereum and donovanosis. Genitourin Med 1992;68:130–133.

MYCOBACTERIAL INFECTIONS

Mycobacteria are thin gram-positive organisms that are obligate aerobes. Because they retain the gram-positive stain despite decolorization with acid-alcohol, they are called *acid-fast bacilli*. They may be categorized according to the diseases they cause: cutaneous tuberculosis, leprosy, and atypical mycobacterial infections or environmental mycobacterial infections. Alternate classifications discuss tuberculosis for those diseases caused by *Mycobacterium tuberculosis* and mycobacterioses for the diseases caused by other mycobacteria. This latter group has been referred to as *mycobacteria other than tuberculosis*, or MOTT.

CUTANEOUS TUBERCULOSIS

In the past, incidences of cutaneous tuberculosis had decreased dramatically, owing to pasteurization of milk, effective antituberculous therapy, and improved living standards. There is now, however, a resurgence worldwide of this disease. The causes are unclear, but immunosuppressed patients have a higher frequency of tubercular infection.

ETIOLOGY

M. tuberculosis causes several different types of cutaneous infection through primary infection of the skin or secondary reaction to internal infection. Some types of cutaneous tuberculosis are considered to reflect id or allergic responses (Table 5). *Mycobacterium bovis* rarely infects humans today, while Bacillus Calmette-Guérin (BCG), although infrequently, creates a cutaneous lesion.

Table 5.1 Types of Cutaneous Tuberculosis

Type	Pathogenesis
primary tuberculosis	
tuberculous chancre	inoculation
miliary tuberculosis	hematogenous
secondary tuberculosis	
acute miliary tuberculosis of the skin	hematogenous
lupus vulgaris	lymphatic or hematogenous
tuberculosis verrucosa cutis	inoculation
scrofuloderma	direct extension from adenitis or bone
tuberculosis cutis orificialis	direct extension from adenitis or bone
tuberculid	
erythema induratum	hematogenous
lichen scrofulosorum	hematogenous
papulonecrotic tuberculid	hematogenous

CLINICAL PRESENTATION

Tuberculous chancre Occurs most often on the face or the extremities, 2 to 3 weeks following inoculation of the tubercle bacillus in a patient with no immunologic recall of prior exposure. The lesion begins as a brownish red papule which becomes a nodule or indurated plaque. Within a month's time, it becomes impetiginized and later ulcerated with heaped-up, ragged borders. The regional lymphadenopathy is prominent (Figure 37a).

BCGitis A variation of the tuberculous chancre. This develops at the site of the BCG vaccination, given as prophylaxis against tuberculosis. Although not commonly done in the United States at present, BCG vaccination is used in the treatment of some malignancies (Figure 37b).

Miliary tuberculosis Occurs in infants, children, or adults who are immunocompromised. There is massive tuberculemia, often following a previously unrelated infection. In addition to such systemic signs as malaise, fever, and night sweats, there are reddish to purplish macules, papules, and vesicles scattered over the body. These cutaneous lesions may ulcerate and even give a gummatous appearance (Figure 37c).

Lupus vulgaris Develops through lymphatic or hematogenous dissemination or as an extension of a primary lesion in an immunocompetent patient who is sensitive to the tubercle bacillus. The characteristic apple-jelly nodules are best seen on diascopy (Figure 37d). Atrophic plaque with an elevated border usually occurs on the head and neck.

Scrofuloderma Begins as a firm reddish brown subcutaneous nodule that evolves into a plaque with a doughy center. The lesion breaks down to form ulcers with a linear or serpiginous shape and undermined borders. Healing occurs with bridging scars. The lesions occurs most often in the submandibular or supraclavicular area or the lateral aspects of the neck (Figure 37e).

Tuberculosis verrucosa cutis A verrucous lesion, usually found on the hands and arms in immunocompetent patients who have had prior exposure to the tubercle bacillus. An erythematous papule or papulopustule is the first sign (prospector's wart). This progresses to a warty lesion with a purplish to brownish base. Satellite lesions develop along with central atrophy and scarring. There is no lymphadenopathy (Figure 37f).

Papulonecrotic tuberculid Often appears on the face as papules that become crusted and necrotic. Because it may resemble acne, it has also been called *acnitis* (Figure 37g). Most believe that acnitis is actually granulomalous rosacea.

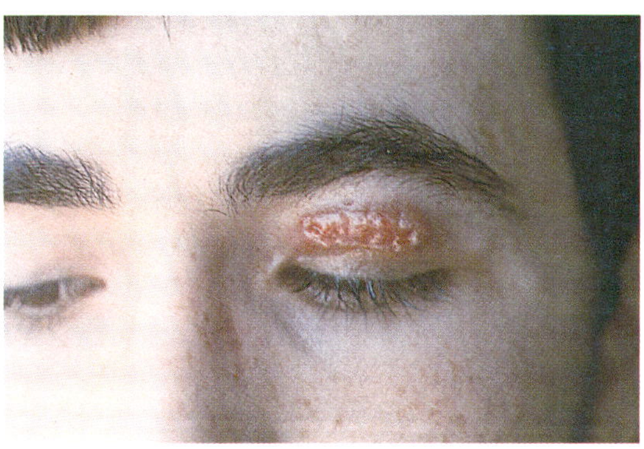

a

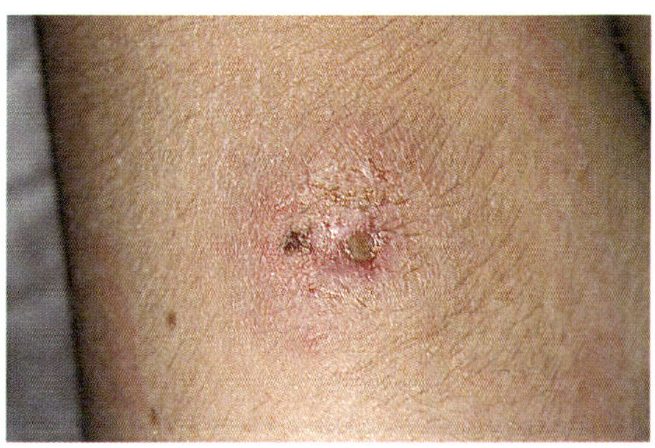

b

Figure 37
(a) Tuberculous chancre represents a firm ulcerated lesion as found on this patient's upper eyelid. (Courtesy of Shukrallah Zaynoun, MD, Beirut, Lebanon.) (b) BCGitis is characterized as a firm, indurated ulcer that develops shortly after the patient received a BCG vaccination. (Courtesy of Guy Chabeau, MD, Lyon, France.) (c) Miliary tuberculosis may be seen as red to purplish papules, scattered on the legs. Some lesions are discrete and others are confluent. (d) Lupus vulgaris was diagnosed when apple jelly nodules were revealed by diascopy. (e) Scrofuloderma shows reddish plaques with some ulcerations. (f) Tuberculosis verrucosa cutis appears as crusted, warty plaques on the body. (Courtesy of Guy Chabeau, MD, Lyon, France.) (g) Papulonecrotic tuberculid appears as papules, some of which may be necrotic (Courtesy of Kyrill Pramatarov, MD, Sofia, Bulgaria.)

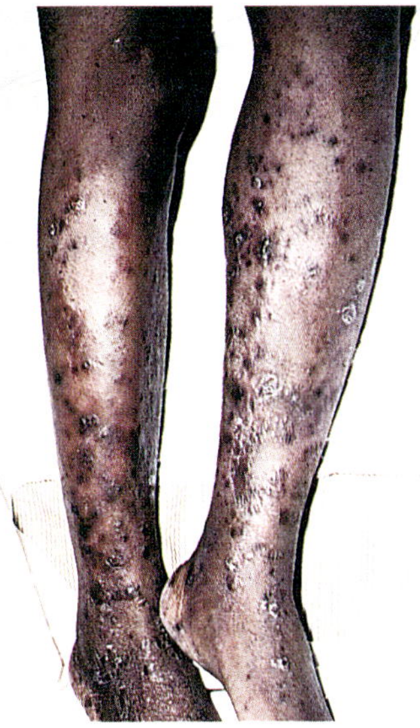

c

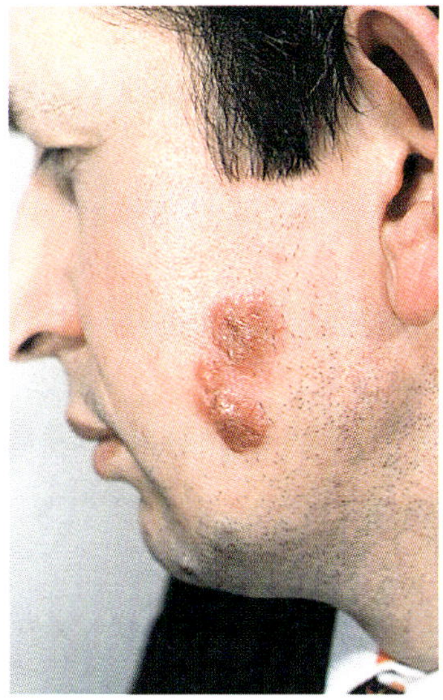

d

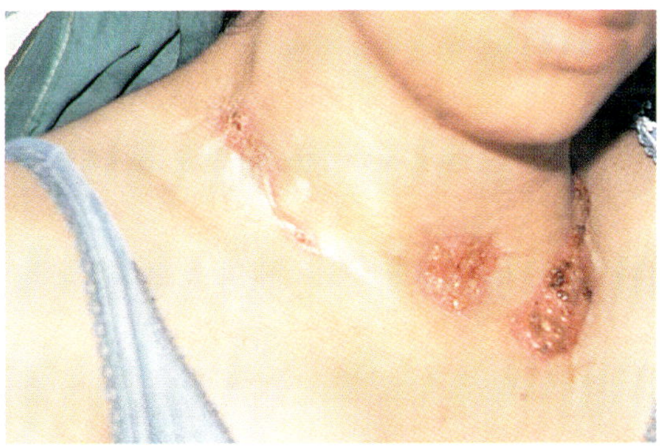

e

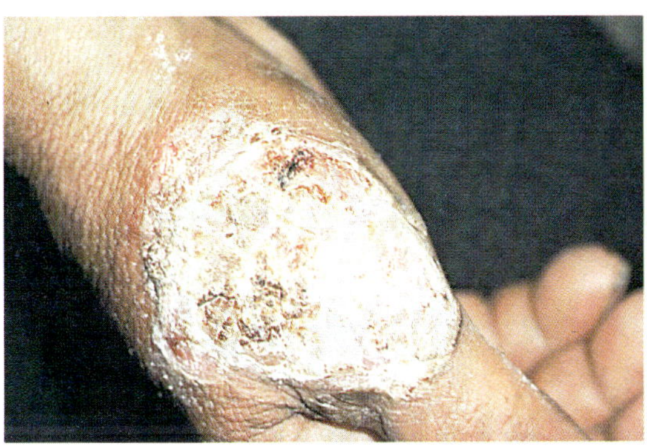

f

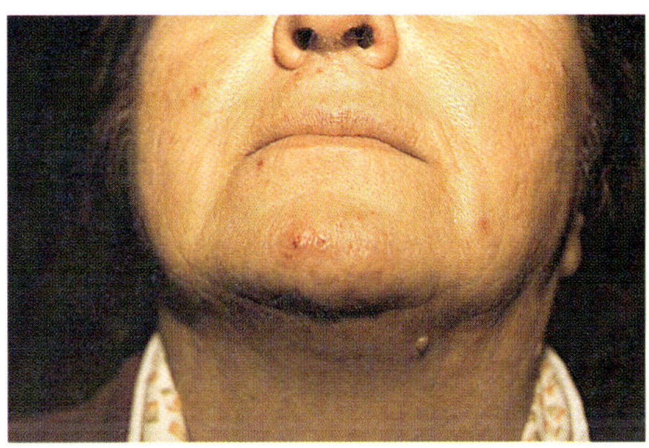

g

DIAGNOSIS

Generally, the diagnosis of cutaneous tuberculosis is made on clinical grounds, especially when suspicion is high. Histopathologic study of a biopsy specimen will generally show a granulomatous process, while special stains may illustrate the acid-fast bacilli. Cultures may also reveal the tubercle bacillus in certain types of cutaneous tuberculosis.

DIFFERENTIAL DIAGNOSIS

The clinical manifestations of cutaneous tuberculosis can be confused with a wide variety of infections, ranging from primary syphilis to deep mycotic infections.

TREATMENT

Triple chemotherapy with isoniazid (5–10 mg/kg/day up to 300 mg/day), rifampin (10–20 mg/kg/day up to 600 mg/day), and ethambutol (15–25 mg/kg/day), pyrazinamide (15–30 mg/kg/day), or streptomycin (15–20 mg/kg/day up to 1 gm/day) is recommended for approximately 9 months. Surgical debridement is sometimes indicated.

SUGGESTED READINGS

Figueriredo A, Poiares-Baptista A, Branco M, et al. Papular tuberculids post-BCG vaccination. Int J Dermatol 1987;26:291–294.

Kakakhel KU, Fritsch P. Cutaneous tuberculosis. Int J Dermatol 1989;28:355–362.

Sehgal VN, Bhattacharya SN, Jain S, Logani K. Cutaneous tuberculosis: the evolving scenario. Int J Dermatol 1994;33:97–104.

Seghal VN, Wagh SA. Cutaneous tuberculosis: current concepts. Int J Dermatol 1990; 29:237–252.

Telenti A, Imboden P, Marchesi F, et al. Detection of rifampicin-resistance mutations in Mycobacterium tuberculosis. Lancet 1993;341:647–650.

Victor T, Jordaan HF, Van Niekerk DJT, et al. Papulonecrotic tuberculid: identification of Mycobacterium tuberculosis DNA by polymerase chain reaction. Am J Dermatopathol 1992;14:491–495.

LEPROSY

Leprosy is a chronic granulomatous infection that is also called *Hansen's disease*. The extent of the devastation caused is related to the immunologic status of the patient, although the mutilations, so well-known from the Middle Ages, are rare today.

ETIOLOGY

The disease is caused by *Mycobacterium leprae*, and the incubation period, still undetermined, may extend up to 20 years. Transmission of the bacilli may be through airborne means to susceptible people.

CLINICAL PRESENTATION

There are four major types of leprosy: tuberculoid, lepromatous, indeterminate, and borderline (dimorphous).

Tuberculoid leprosy Distinguished by a good immunologic response. The lepromin skin test is positive, with few bacilli found in the tissue. The lesions are few in number, assymmetrical, and hypopigmented to red macules or patches with a well-defined border. An enlarged peripheral nerve may be palpable at the edge of the lesion. The lesion is often anesthetic (Figure 38a).

Lepromatous leprosy Characterized by diffuse and widespread, normal skin colored to red macules, papules, plaques, and nodules. The lesions are bilateral and symmetrical, frequently found on the earlobes, face, arms, and buttocks. There are numerous bacilli seen on histologic sections, and the lepromin test is negative. The immunologic status of the patient is compromised (Figure 38b).

Borderline leprosy (dimorphous) Representative of features of both the tuberculoid and lepromatous types. This results because the body cannot determine the immunologic response and vacillates between each major type. The lesions are multiple and asymmetric, but there are well-defined macules or papules and sometimes nodules or plaques. There may be little or no sensory loss to complete anethesia of the lesions. Bacilli are found on smear. The lepromin skin test may be either weakly positive or negative (Figure 38c,d).

Indeterminate leprosy Distinguished by ill-defined lesions that may be erythematous or hypopigmented macules and borders that are usually vague. The lesions may be found alone or in mutiple asymmetric groups. Sensation is normal or slightly impaired. No bacilli are found on smear. The lepromin test may be either negative or positive.

DIAGNOSIS

The clinical picture is often suggestive, but histologic examination will frequently support the diagnosis. Depending upon the type of leprosy, lepra bacilli can be seen, particularly when the tissue is stained with Fite's.

DIFFERENTIAL DIAGNOSIS

Leprosy can be confused with many diagnoses, ranging from vitiligo to a deep mycotic infection or even a malignancy.

TREATMENT

Dapsone, 100 mg/day is given for several years, along with rifampicin, 600 mg monthly, for 6 months. The addition of cimetidine, 400 mg tid may reduce the methemoglobinemia that occurs in some patients. Depending on the type of leprosy, clofazimine, 50 mg/day, or rifampin, 600 mg/day, may be used. Clarithromycin, 500 mg daily may also be added to the regimen.

SUGGESTED READINGS

Britton WJ. Leprosy 1962–1992: 3. Immunology of leprosy. Trans Roy Soc Trop Med Hyg 1993;87:508–514.

Bryceson A, Pfaltzgradd RE. Leprosy. New York, Churchill Livingstone, 1990:1–240.

Okoro AN. Pre-emptive diagnosis of leprosy. Int J Dermatol 1991;30:767–771.

Ross M, Barr RJ. Leprosy in the United States: just a curiosity? Int J Dermatol 1991;30:772–773.

Sehgal VN, Joginder, Sharma VK. Immunology of leprosy: a comprehensive survey. Int J Dermatol 1989;28:574–584.

Sehgal VN, Leprosy. Dermatol Clin 1994;12:629–644.

Waters MFR. Leprosy 1962-1993: 1. Chemo-therapy of leprosy–current status and future prospects. Trans Roy Soc Trop Med 1993; 87:500–503.

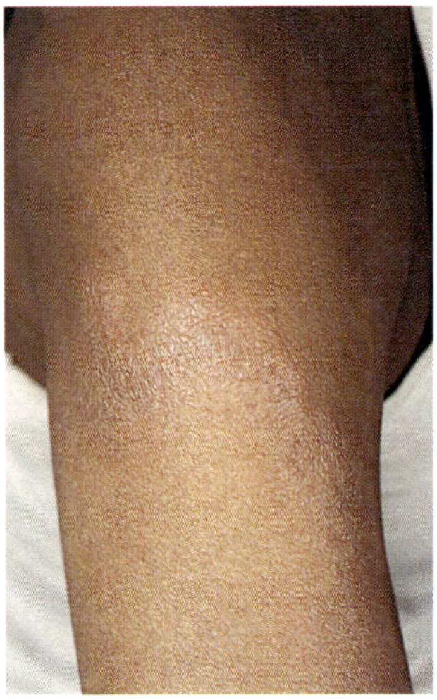

a

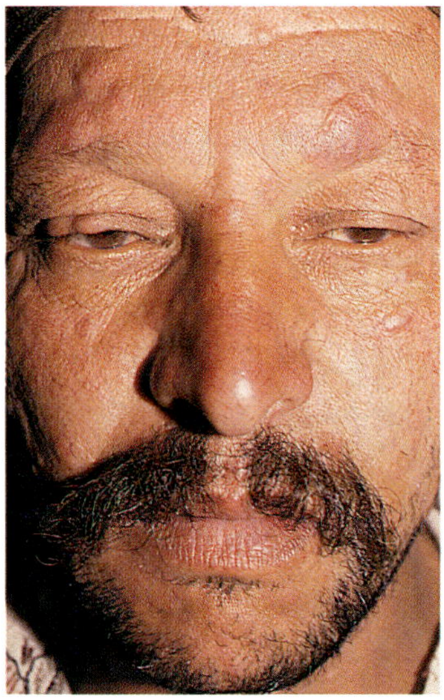

b

Figure 38
(a) Tuberculoid leprosy is characterized by hypopigmented, scaling patches. (Courtesy of Qasem A. Alsaleh, MD, Kuwait City, Kuwait.) (b) Lepromatous leprosy, as seen in this Tunisian man, has purplish areas with less distinct borders. (Courtesy of Selim Zahaf, MD, Sfax, Tunisia.) (c) Borderline leprosy was diagnosed in this 22-year-old woman who presented to the Vargas Hospital in Caracas, Venezuela. The lesion contained a darker, nodular area. (d) Indeterminate leprosy may present as a nonspecific dermatitis with some scaling and lightening of the skin. (Courtesy of Béatrice Flageul, MD, Paris, France.)

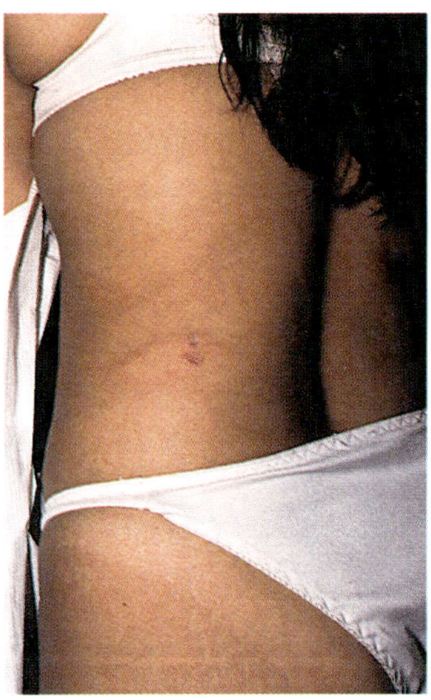

c

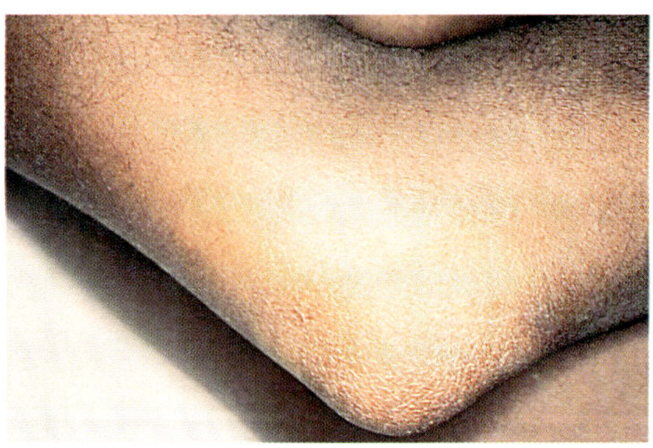

d

Atypical Mycobacterial Infections

Atypical mycobacterial infections of the skin have increased in frequency in recent years due in part to the increase in invasive procedures, intravenous drug addiction, and the number of patients with decreased immunity. Steroid injections, both intradermally and intramuscularly, have occasionally resulted in infections.

ETIOLOGY

The atypical mycobacteria are usually commensals or saprophytes but under certain conditions become pathogenic to humans. They have been classified according to their growth patterns and the influence of light on their characteristics (Table 6). More than 50 species have been identified, of which nearly half are pathogenic for humans. Those organisms which have a significant propensity for the skin include: *M. avium-intracellulare*, *M. chelonei*, *M. fortuitum*, *M. marinum*, *M. smegmatis*, and *M. ulcerans*.

Table 6 Atypical Mycobacteria

A. Slow growers (2-3 week requirement)	
Group I	
Photochromogens	*M. marinum* (yellow color on light exposure)
	M. kansasii
	M. simiae
Group II	
Scotochromogens	*M. scrofulaceum* (yellow color even without light exposure)
	M. flavescens
	M. azulgai
Group III	
Non-chromogens	*M. avium-intracellulare*
	M. gastrii
	M. terrae
	M. triviale
	M. xenopi
	M. haemophilum
	M. novum
	M. chromogenicum
B. Rapid growers (3 to 5 day requirement)	
Group IV	
Rapid growers	*M. fortuitum*
	M. chelonei
	M. phlei
	M. vaccae
	M. smegmatis
	M. diernhoferi

Adapted from: Lotti T, Hautmann G. Atypical mycobacterial infections: A difficult and emerging group of infectious dermatoses. Int J Dermatol 1993;32:499-501.

CLINICAL PRESENTATION

Buruli ulcer Caused by *M. ulcerans,* occurs most often in Africa, although it was first recognized in Australia (Bairnsdale ulcer). It is characterized by single or multiple ulcerations that range in size from a few millimeters to several centimeters. There are undermined borders, and the base of the ulcer contains an adherent grayish pseudomembrane. The ulcer or ulcers can enlarge enough on an extremity to require amputation, although spontaneous regression is known (Figure 39a). The lesion is painless and the patient feels well.

Swimming pool granuloma Caused by *M. marinum,* and is traditionally is found in fishermen or patients cleaning fish tanks or swimming pools. When the skin is traumatized, the bacterium can penetrate. Within a 2 to 6 week period following the injury, red papules appear that form nontender purplish nodules which may crust and ulcerate. The lesions are generally localized to the hands, feet, elbows, and knees. Occasionally, lesions develop along a lymphatic vessel or an extremity (sporatrichera pattern) and are found on the arm, resemble sporotrichosis, and may spontaneously regress in months or even years (Figure 39b).

Abscess formation Caused by *M. fortuitum, M. chelonei,* and *M. smegmatis.* Abscesses often develop very subtly. The initiating factor may be trauma, surgical intervention, or even injections with contaminated materials. Within a 4 to 6 week period, but for as long as a year, the area becomes inflamed with development of an abscess. Lymphadenopathy and systemic signs of infection may occur (Figure 39c).

Sporotrichoid cutaneous infection Caused by *M. kansasii* or *M. chelonei* , presents itself as a chronic granulomatous disease, usually in association with chronic pulmonary infection. The skin manifestation appears to be caused by extension or metastasis from the internal infection. Sometimes, the infection created by this atypical mycobacterium becomes ulcerated or presents as cellulitis or pyoderma (Figure 39d).

M. avium-intracellulare infection May have many varied clinical manifestations ranging from papules and nodules to ulcers overlying infected bone or lymph nodes. Rosacea has even been reported (Figure 39e).

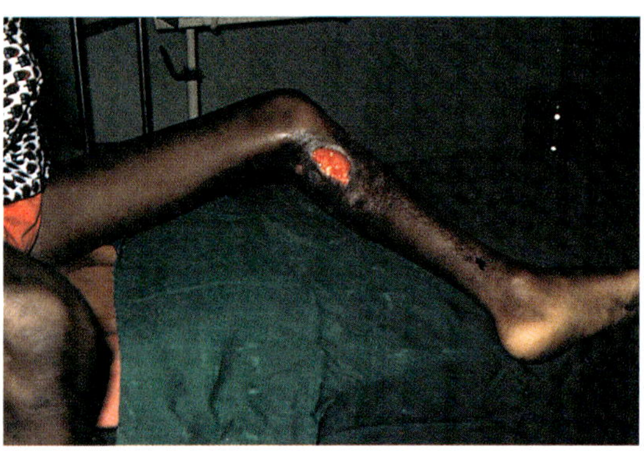

a

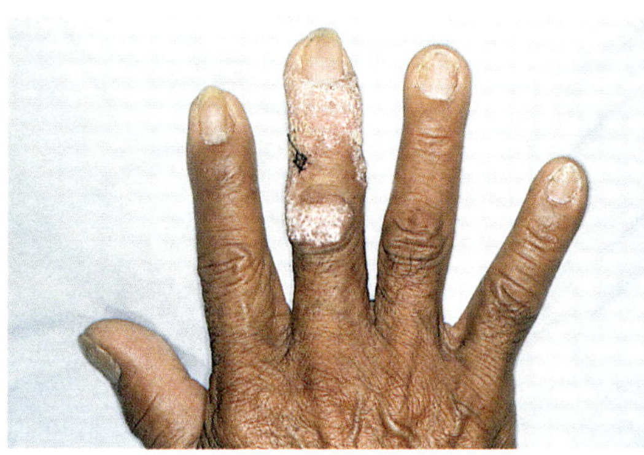

b

Figure 39
(a) Buruli ulcer was diagnosed in this African patient, when *M. ulcerans* was recovered from his ragged, crusted ulcer. (Courtesy of Wolfram Höffler, MD, Tübingen, Germany.) (b) Swimming pool granuloma is a hyperkeratotic, scaling plaque. (Courtesy of R. Ismael, MD, Kuala Lumpur, Malaysia.) (c) Abscess formation in this patient might appear to be due to pyogenic bacteria; however, the physician was eventually able to culture out *M. chelonae*. (Courtesy of Roberto Arenas, MD, Mexico City, Mexico.) (d) This organism can also create a sporotrichoid pattern. (Courtesy of Kenneth Greer, MD, Charlottesville, VA.) (e) In *M. avium-intracellulare* , there may be an erythematous papular eruption that resembles rosacea.

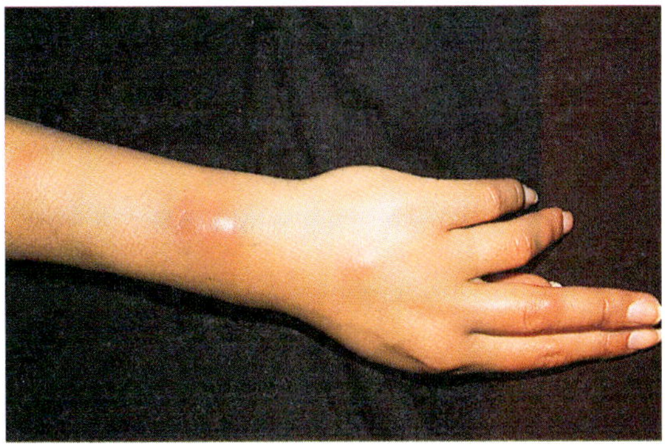

c

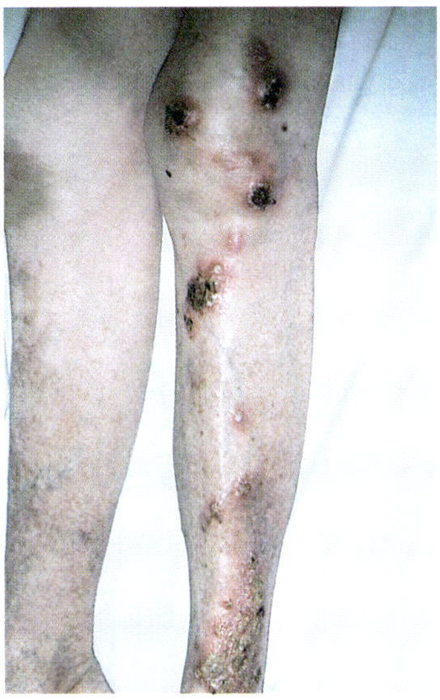

d

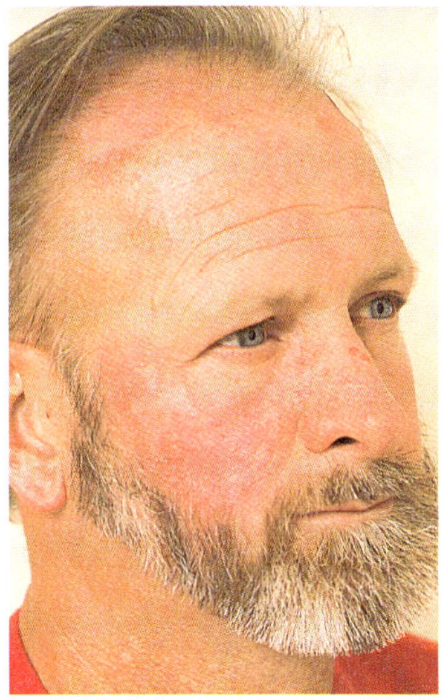

e

DIAGNOSIS

Culture of the drainage or of a biopsy specimen will reveal the pathogen. The laboratory must be instructed that a mycobacterium is suspected, so that incubation temperatures can be adjusted.

DIFFERENTIAL DIAGNOSIS

The lesions are often confused with ulcers of other causes or with the cutaneous manifestations of deep fungal infections. Occasionally, viral infections, such as those caused by the papillomavirus, can have similar presentations.

TREATMENT

Each of these organisms has variable sensitivities to antimicrobial agents. Usually, rifampin, 600 mg/day, ciprofloxacin, 750 mg bid, tetracycline, 1 gm/day, clofazamine, 200mg/day, or clarithromycin, 250 mg qid, given for several weeks, is curative. Triple antimicrobial therapy often may be required.

SUGGESTED READINGS

Bonafe JL, Larrue N. Atypical cutaneous mycobacterial infections. Nouv Dermatol 1994;13:63–69.

Greer KE, Gross GP, Martensen SH. Sporotrichoid cutaneous infection due to Mycobacterium chelonei. Arch Dermatol 1979;115:738–739.

Kullavanijaya P, Sirimachan S, Bhuddhavudhikrai P. Mycobacterium marinum infections acquired from occupations and hobbies. Int J Dermatol 1993;32:504–507.

Lotti T, Hautmann G. Atypical mycobacterial infections: A difficult and emerging group of infectious dermatoses. Int J Dermatol 1993:32:499–501.

Nedorost ST, Elewski B, Tomford JW, et al. Rosacea-like lesions due to familial Mycobacterium avium-intracellulare infection. Int J Dermatol 1991;30:491–497.

Ribera M, Bielsa J, Manterola JM, et al. *Mycobacterium boris*–BCG infection of the glans penis: complication of intravesical administration of bacillus Calmette-Guerin. Br J Dermatol 1995;132:309–310.

Rotman DA, Blauvelt A, Kerdel FA. Widespread primary infection with Mycobacterium fortuitum. Int J Dermatol 1993;32:512–516.

Stark JR. Nontuberculous mycobacterial infections in children. Adv Ped Infect Dis 1992;7:123-159.

Street ML, Umbert-Millet IJ, Roberts GD, et al Nontuberculous mycobacterial infections of the skin. J Am Acad Dermatol 1991;24:208–215

SPIROCHETAL INFECTIONS

The treponemes are members of the Spirochaetales order. Because of their generally small size (10–13μ x 0.15μ) they cannot be visualized by light microscopy. The advent of the dark-field microscope helped to identify their corkscrew shape and their motility. These organisms can not be readily grown in vitro.

In addition to causing syphilis, spirochetes are the agents of yaws, bejel, pinta, relapsing fever, and lyme borreliosis. Possibly, the causative organisms evolved from the same treponeme, but conclusive evidence is not available.

SYPHILIS

Syphilis has so many different manifestations that Sir William Osler once remarked that to know syphilis is to know medicine.

ETIOLOGY

Treponema pallidum is the pathogen. Finding animal models has been difficult. Under some circumstances, the organism will grow in hamsters, guinea pigs, and mice. It is pathogenic for anthropoid apes and rabbits. Syphilis is most often transmitted by personal contact with an infectious person; however, patients have been infected through blood transfusions or even from contaminated drinking cups.

CLINICAL PRESENTATION

Syphilis can be divided into three stages. In the *primary* stage, within 9 to 90 days after exposure, a painless ulcer appears at the point of contact. This is usually found on the genitalia, but it can be located anywhere on the body. The ulcer or chancre begins as a painless, erythematous papule or crusted erosion that becomes an indurated, round or oval ulcer. The accompanying regional lymphadenopathy is usually bilateral and painless. If the lesion becomes secondarily infected, some pain might be noted. The chancre clears in 3 to 8 weeks, generally without scarring (Figure 40a,b).

Sometime between 1 and 20 weeks after the clearing of the chancre, *secondary* lesions appear along with flu-like symptoms—myalgia, malaise, headache, arthralgia, rhinorrhea, and fever. The most characteristic lesions are the coppery or raw ham-colored macules on the palms and soles. Macular and papular, pink to copper-colored lesions can also be found elsewhere on the body. Other lesions, ranging from psoriasiform to hypopigmented macules, may appear. There may be a succession of conspicuously generalized eruptions. Pruritus is usually limited to black patients. Patchy alopecia ("moth-eaten alopecia") may be present, along with an injected pharynx and red papules covered with grayish exudate on the mucosal surfaces. These findings disappear within several weeks, regardless of treatment (Figure 40c,d,e). Generalized lymphadenopathy is usually present.

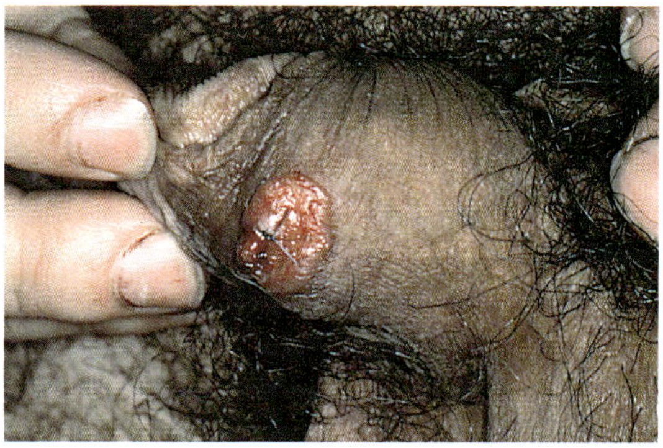

a

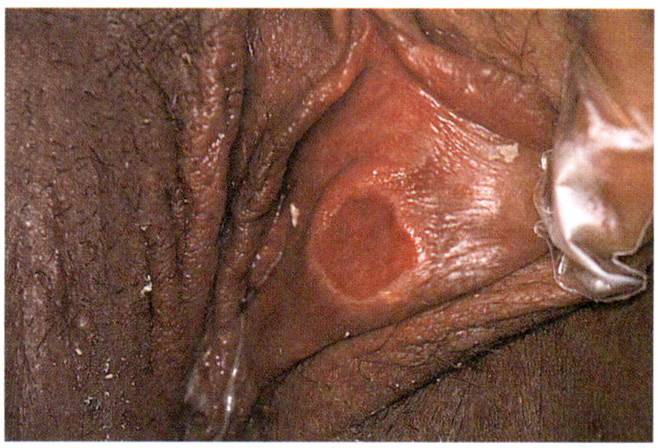

b

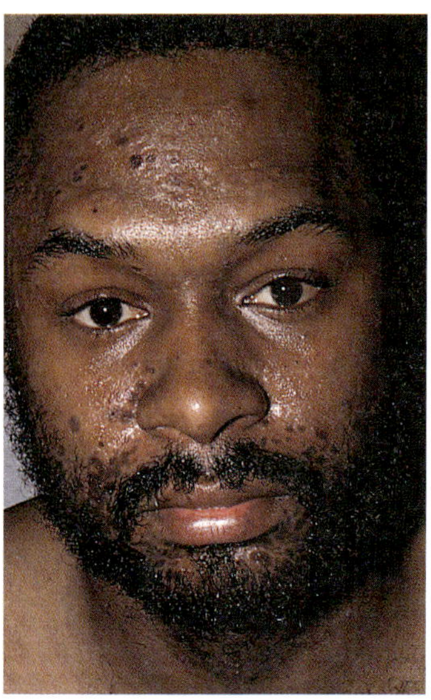

c

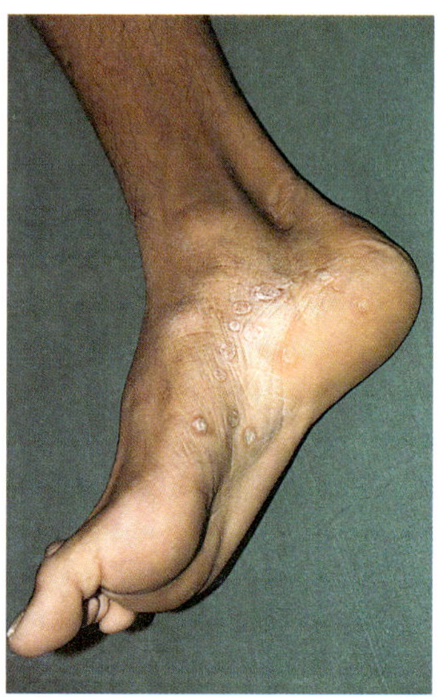

d

Figure 40
Syphilis appears as an eroded, indurated plaque or hard chancre in the primary stage. (a) Penile and (b) labial ulcerations are common locations. (Courtesy of Selim Aractingi, MD, Paris, France.) The diagnosis of the secondary stage of syphilis is often made by finding a diffuse eruption of erythematous macules. (c) The first patient has the characteristic copper-colored macules coupled with purplish to necrotic papules. (d) The second patient has the macular lesions on the feet, where there is peripheral scaling. (Courtesy of Michel Janvier, MD, Paris, France.) (e) Pityriasis rosea may be distinguished by the oval lesions that often have central scaling, rather than the peripheral scaling of secondary syphilis, plus the herald patch, pruritus, and lack of lymphadenopathy. The tertiary stage of syphilis is characterized by gummas that may be localized as shown in the first patient (f). They may also be more diffuse and demonstrate extensive destruction (g). (Courtesy of the Bertram Shaffer, MD Collection of the College of Physicians of Philadelphia.) Congenital syphilis appears as (h) snuffles in infancy. This baby also had perioral erosions and crusting. If the infection is untreated, interference with dental development leads to (i) defective tooth formation (Hutchinson's teeth). (Courtesy of Esther Wakszol de Schmidmajer, MD, Caracas, Venezuela.)

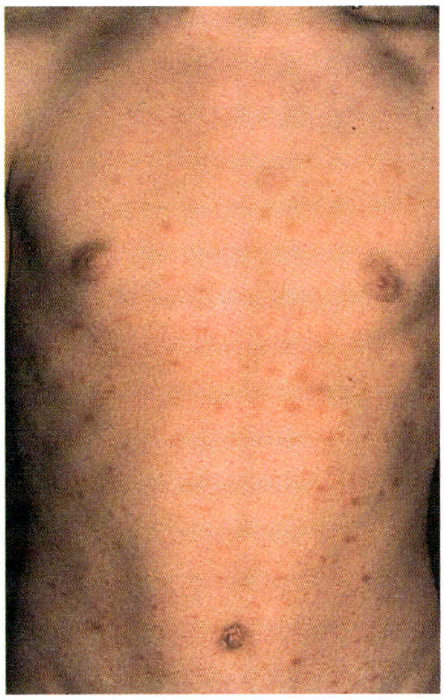

e

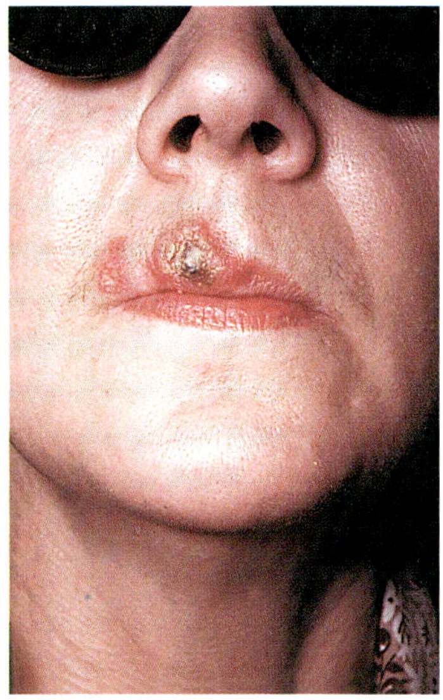

f

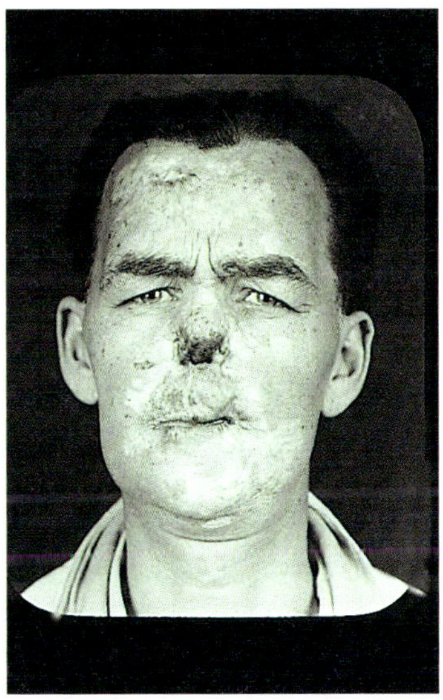

g

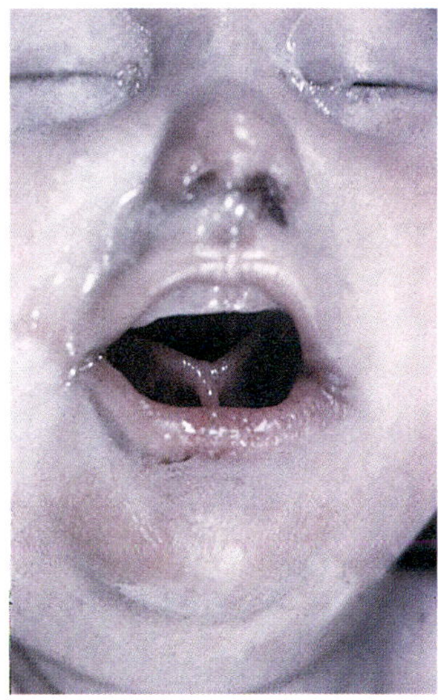

h

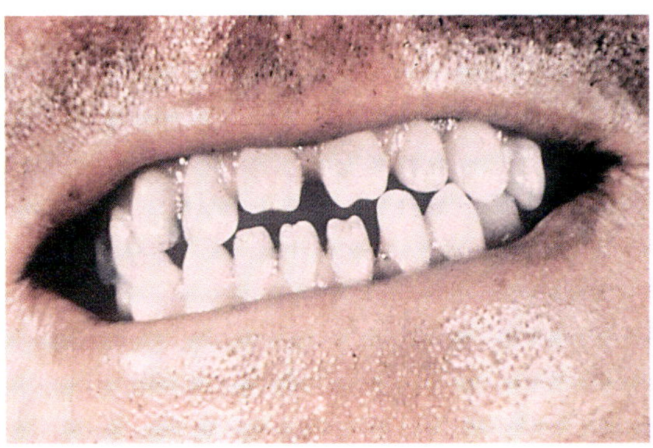

i

In the *tertiary* stage, the early latent phase lasts for 2 years and shows no recognizable signs. Occasionally, a gumma, which is an erythematous nodule that ulcerates and contains a grayish membrane and discharges gummy material, may develop early (Figure 40f).

There are no signs or symptoms during the latent stage. The tertiary stage occurs 3 to 15 years after the primary stage; two types of mucocutaneous lesions manifest—nodular or nodula-ulcerative and gummatous. In addition to heart disease, dementia (general paresis, neurologic damage), and tabes dorsalis, there is destruction of joints (Charcot's joint)(Figure 40g).

Congenital syphilis , once known as syphilis of the innocent, is characterized by a wizened appearance in young children. The newborn may have bullous lesions, snuffles, and rhinitis with painful periostitis and osteochondritis (Figure 40h) Eventually, the untreated patient may have Hutchinson's triad: mulberry molars, interstitial keratitis, and neural deafness, as well as hydroarthrosis (Clutton's joint), frontal bossing, and saddle nose (Figure 40j).

DIAGNOSIS

The clinical findings can be confirmed by finding *T. pallidum* in a dark-field smear taken from a moist lesion of the primary and early secondary stages. The serologic tests will usually be reactive by the beginning of the secondary stage, although patients with human immunodeficiency virus (HIV) infection may not have elevated titers or even reactive serologies.

DIFFERENTIAL DIAGNOSIS

The chancre may be confused with other types of genital ulcers such as chancroid, herpes progenitalis, or a pyogenic ulcer. The secondary stage may resemble pityriasis rosea, erythema multiforme, or a drug eruption. The tertiary stage may resemble one of the connective tissue diseases.

TREATMENT

Benzathine penicillin, 2.4 million units, is given once for primary syphilis, repeated in 1 week for secondary syphilis, and repeated again in a week for tertiary syphilis. Penicillin-sensitive patients may be given erythromycin or tetracycline, 500 mg qid, for 15 days. Cephalosporins may also be used, although the quinolones have no antisyphilitic activity.

SUGGESTED READINGS

Crissey JT, Denenholtz DA. Syphilis. Clin Dermatol 1984;2(1)1-166.

Engelkens HJH. Syphilis and the endemic treponematoses. Rotterdam, Erasmus University. 1993:1-208.

Johnson PC, Farnie MA. Testing for syphilis. Dermatol Clin 1994;12:9–17.

Lowy G. Sexually transmitted diseases in children. Ped Dermatol 1992;9:329–334.

Tosca A, Stavropoulos PG, Hatzlolu E, et al. Malignant syphilis in HIV-infected patients. Int J Dermatol 1990;29:575–578.

Willcox RR. The treponemal evolution. Trans St. John's Hosp Dermatol Soc 1972;58:21–37.

Endemic treponematoses

Endemic treponematoses were almost eradicated in the 1950s and 1960s through widespread penicillin therapy under the direction of the World Health Organization. Unfortunately, there are now resurgences of yaws (framboesia tropica, pian, buba) in many parts of Africa; of endemic syiphilis (bejel, treponarid) in the hot, dry areas of Africa, western Asia, and Australia; and of pinta (mal del pinto) in Central and South America.

ETIOLOGY

Treponema pertenue (yaws) cannot be distinguished from *T. pallidum* (syphilis), *T. pallidum endemicum* (endemic syphilis [bejel]), or *T. carateum* (pinta); however, *T. pertenue* can be passed through rabbits and hamsters.

CLINICAL PRESENTATION

Yaws is divided into three stages. In the primary stage, 9 to 90 days after infection, the mother yaw develops. This is a nontender papule that may become crusted and ulcerated, usually occurring on the leg at the site of inoculation (Figure 41a). In the secondary stage, the lesion disappears only to reappear (daughter yaws) with accompanying malaise and systemic distress. These lesions are multiple and smaller, found on the face and extremities, and are soft, raspberry-like, granulomatous lesions (Figure 41b).

After an indeterminate period of latency (the tertiary stage) during which there may be relapses, late yaws develops. These destructive lesions include hyperkeratotic skin lesions, exostoses of the nose or bone (gondou), and ulceration and destruction of the nose and pharynx (gangosa). Many late lesions also mimic syphilis (Figure 41c).

Endemic syphilis presents a clinical picture very much like the one found in yaws; however, the disease is not transmitted sexually. There are three stages beginning with a chancre, which is rarely recognized, progressing to mucous membrane lesions and a maculopapular eruption and, finally, revealing gummas and bone changes (Figure 42). Endemic syphilis, like syphilis, mimics many diseases including psoriasis, viral infections, and drug eruptions.

Pinta is a cutaneous malady with three stages. Initially, there are plaques on the extremities. These are red, scaling plaques that enlarge. Three to 6 months later, erythematosquamous patches develop on much of the body. In the tertiary stage, which occurs 2 to 5 years later, there are pigmented areas that range from gray or ashy to steel or dark blue. These become achromic (Figure 43). Pinta can be confused with dermatophytosis, psoriasis, erythema dyschromicum perstans, or vitiligo.

DIAGNOSIS

As in syphilis, a dark-field examination in the early, infectious stages will confirm the clinical impression. In later stages, the serologic tests for syphilis will be reactive. A biopsy of the lesion will show, on histopathologic examination, plasma cells in the dense dermal inflammatory infiltrate and epidermal hyperplasia. With a silver stain, the organism can be seen in the early stages.

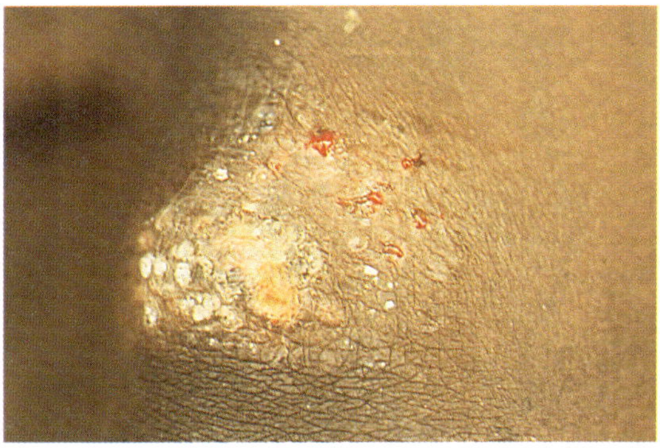

a

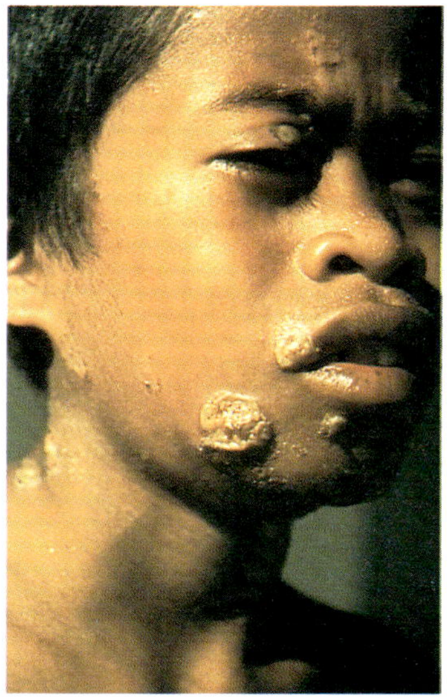

b

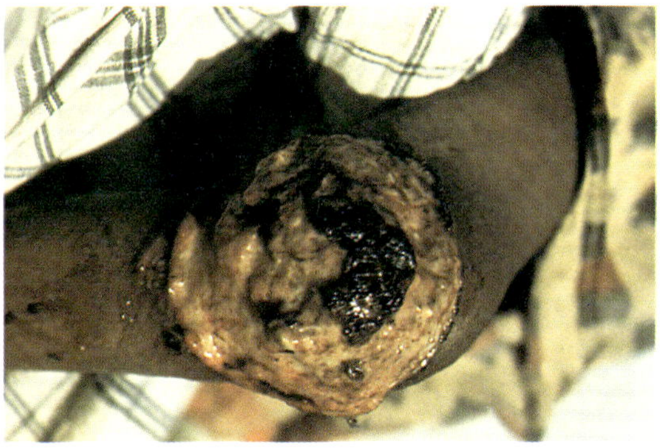

c

Figure 41
Yaws initially appears (a) as an isolated crusted lesion at the site of inoculation or later (b) as several lesions with the so-called mother and daughter lesions. In the late stage, (c) the gumma is shown as a purulent, crusted ulceration. (Courtesy of Wolfram Höffler, MD, Tübingen, Germany.)

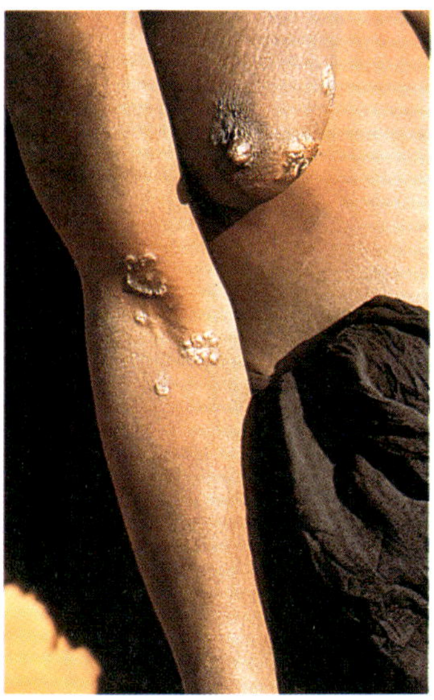

Figure 42
The secondary lesions of endemic syphilis are papular, annular, and crusted. (Courtesy of Wolfram Höffler, MD, Tübingen, Germany.)

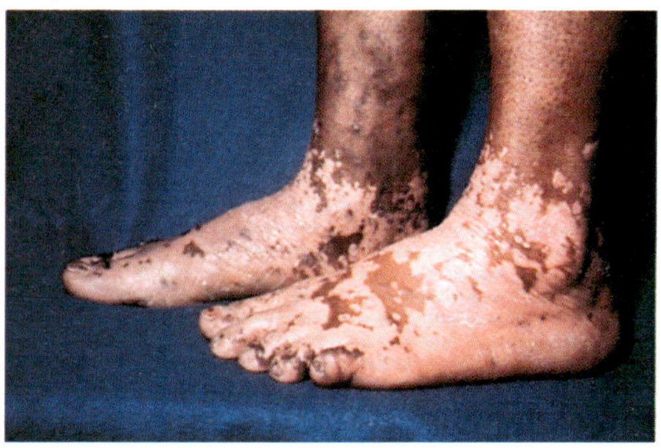

Figure 43
Pinta, as it progresses, leads to hypopigmentation with scaling and slight atrophy. (Courtesy of Antar Padilha-Gonçalves, MD, Rio de Janeiro, Brazil.)

DIFFERENTIAL DIAGNOSIS

Yaws may be confused with pyogenic infections, scabies, and deep mycotic infections. In endemic regions, psoriasis, verrucae, and molluscum contagiosum may be confused with this treponemal infection. Dark-field examination, serologic testing, and a biopsy will differentiate the various diseases.

TREATMENT

Penicillin, erythromycin, or tetracycline is recommended, utilizing the same schedules employed for treating syphilis.

SUGGESTED READINGS

Engelkens HJH, Judanaarso J, Oranje AP, et al. Endemic treponematoses: part I. yaws. Int J Dermatol 1991;30:77–83.

Engelkens HJH, Niemel PLA, van der Sluis JJ, et al. The resurgence of yaws: world-wide consequences. Int J Dermatol 1991;30:99–101.

Engelkens HJH, Niemel PLA, van der Sluis JJ, et al. Endemic treponematoses: Part II. pinta and endemic syphilis. Int J Dermatol 1991;30:231–238.

Freedman D. Sexually transmitted diseases from the tropics: an overview. Dermatol Clin 1994;12:737–746.

Luger AFH. Endemic treponematoses. In Parish LC, Gschnait F, eds. Sexually transmitted diseases: a guide for clinicians. New York: Springer-Verlag, 1989:32–58.

Seghal VN. Leg ulcers caused by yaws and endemic syphilis. Clin Dermatol 1990;8(3&4):166–174.

Tabbara KF. Endemic syphilis (Bejel). Int Ophthalmol 1990;14:379–381.

LYME BORRELIOSIS

Lyme borreliosis had been recognized in retrospect since 1909, when erythema migrans was first described. It is a cutaneous disease with both immediate and delayed systemic manifestations.

ETIOLOGY

Borrelia burgdorferi is transmitted by hard-bodied ticks, usually of the Ixodes family. *B. burgdorferi* includes *B. Burgdorferi* (sensu stricto), *B. garini*, and *B. afzeli*. Although the original cases of lyme disease were recognized in southern New England (Lyme, Connecticut), Lyme disease is found in most of North America and many parts of Europe; in fact, it has global distribution. The organism has a natural reservoir in small rodents. The tick bites this animal and carries it to larger animals such as the white-tail deer. The tick bites again and moves the bacterium to humans.

CLINICAL PRESENTATION

Lyme borreliosis can be divided into three stages.

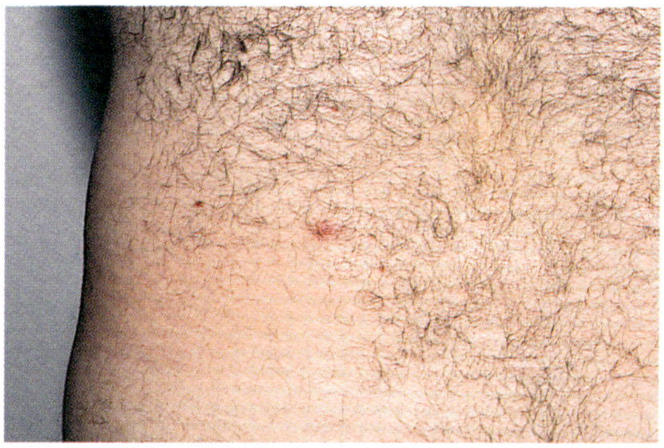

a

Figure 44
Lyme borreliosis begins with (a) a tick bite. Within 3 weeks, the characteristic reddish rings of (b) erythema migrans appear. Later stages include (c) atrophic dermatitis on the hands or feet (acrodermatitis chronica atrophicans) (Courtesy of Antar Padilha-Gonçalves, MD, Rio de Janeiro, Brazil) and (d) a reddish infiltrate on the ear lobes (lymphocytoma benigna). (Courtesy of Carmelo Scarpa, MD, Trieste, Italy.)

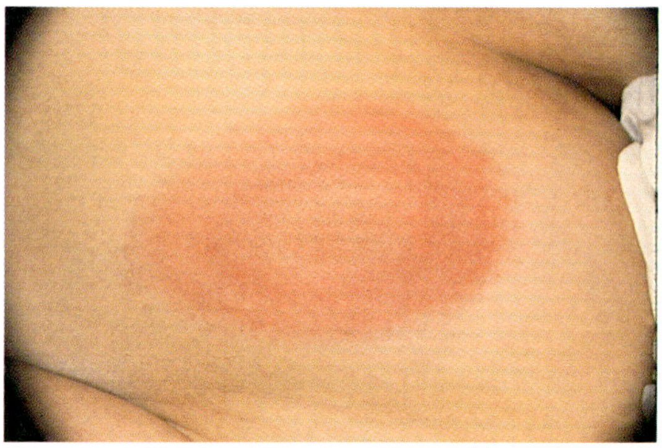

b

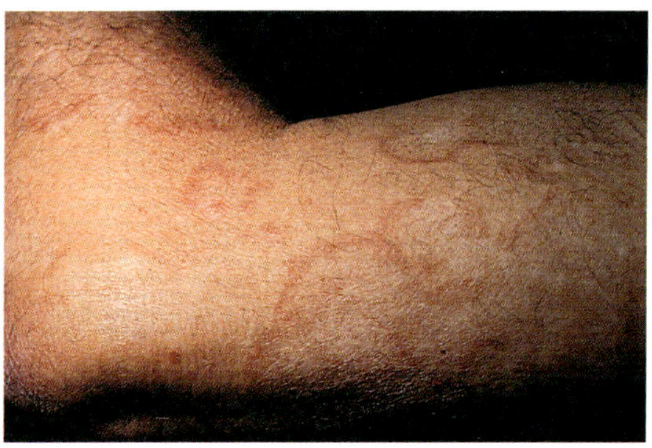

c

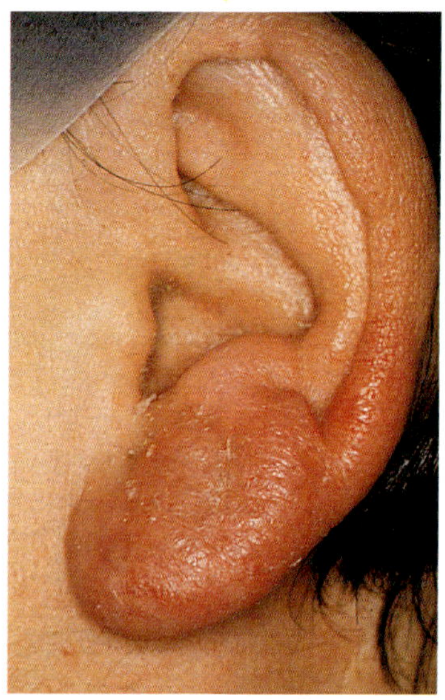

d

Primary Two to 3 weeks following a tick bite, erythema migrans develops (Figure 44a). This is an erythematous lesion with central clearing (Figures 44 b). The patient may also have malaise, headache, and a stiff neck, along with malar flushing and urticaria. Borrelial lymphocytoma is an early manisfestation of Lyme disease.

Secondary Several months later, heart block or aseptic meningitis may occur. A variety of other internal manifestations and malaise develop that may last for several months but are rarely permanent. These include facial palsy, myocarditis, transient arthritis, and iritis. The skin lesions include erythema palmaris and lymphadenosis benigna cutis.

Tertiary Anytime from weeks to months or even years after the initial tick bite, the late manifestations appear. These include arthritis, multiple sclerosis-like disease, and chronic cardiac problems. In Europe and South America, acrodermatitis chronica atrophicans (Figure 44c), a morphea-like disease (Figure 44d) may develop.

DIAGNOSIS

The clinical manifestations may be supported by a biopsy for histopathologic confirmation or by blood tests to detect antibodies against *B. burgdorfei*. These include the indirect immunofluorescence assay (IFA) and enzyme-linked immunosorbent assay (ELISA).

DIFFERENTIAL DIAGNOSIS

In the early stages, tinea corporis, erythema multiforme, or cellulitis may be confused with Lyme borreliosis. Later, rheumatoid arthritis and Guillain-Barré syndrome may be considered.

TREATMENT

In the early phases, amoxicillin, 500 mg tid, doxycycline,100 mg tid,or erythromycin, 250 mg qid, may be given for 3 weeks. Clarithromycin, 250 mg bid, given for 3 weeks is also useful. In more disseminated disease, ceftriaxone, 2 gm/day or penicillin, 4 million units q4h, may be given for 14 to 21 days.

SUGGESTED READINGS

Åsbrink E, Hovmark A. Lyme borreliosis. Clin Dermatol 1993;11:329–429.

Berger BW. Laboratory tests for Lyme disease. Dermatol Clin 1994;12:19–24.

Melski JW. Lyme borreliosis. Fitzpatrick's J Clin Dermatol 1994; 1 (May/June): 14–24.

Pfister H-W, Wilske B, Weber K. Lyme borreliosis: basic science and clinical aspects. Lancet 1994;343:1013–1016.

Scarpa C, Trevisan G, Stinco G: Lyme borreliosis. Dermatol Clin 1994;12:669–686.

Spach DH, Liles WC, Campbell GR, et al. Tick-borne diseases in the United States. N Engl J Med 1993;329:936–947.

Weber K. Clinical management of Lyme borreliosis. Lancet 1994;343:1017–1020.

RICKETTSIACEAE

Rickettsiaceae are small intracellular bacteria that appear as gram negative coccobacilli. They generally are transmitted by arthropods and measure 0.5 μ x 0.3 μ. They contain both deoxyribonucleic acid (DNA) and ribonucleic acid (RNA) and reproduce by binary fission. There are five genera: Rickettsia, Rochalimaea, Coxiella, Ehrlichia, and Bartonella.

RICKETTSIAL INFECTIONS

Of all the infectious diseases, the rickettsial diseases may have the most confusing cutaneous expressions. For the most part, there is an eschar, followed by a maculopapular eruption and in some instances a petechial eruption.

Rocky Mountain Spotted Fever

Rocky Mountain spotted fever is a maculopapular eruption that appears predominantly in the United States in the Rocky Mountain area and the southeast. It has also been found in parts of Mexico and Central and South America.

ETIOLOGY

Rickettsia ricksettsii is transmitted among ticks either transovarially or indirectly by feeding on infected mammals. *Dermacenter andersoni*, the wood tick, spreads the disease in the Rocky Mountains, whereas *D. variablie*, the dog tick, is the vector on the East Coast. Most cases occur from April through August.

CLINICAL PRESENTATION

The disease begins as erythema or a maculopapular eruption on the cooler parts of the body (i.e., palms, soles, male genitalia) and spreads to the trunk, finally becoming generalized (Figure 45a). Early on, there may be high fever, severe headache, and marked myalgias. Nausea, vomiting, diarrhea, and abdominal pain may appear along with the skin findings. A second eruption begins during the second week and is first petechial and and later ecchymotic (Figure 45b). The cutaneous manifestations are subdued or even absent in 15% of the patients, making the clinical presentation confusing. The fatality rate reaches 25% in untreated patients.

DIAGNOSIS

The diagnosis is made clinically, and immunofluorescence studies will reveal the organism. Indirect hemagglutination serologic studies and the Weil-Felix test (agglutination of *Proteus vulgaris* strain [OX-19]) will also assist in making a diagnosis. A cutaneous biopsy may also be needed for the diagnostic workup.

DIFFERENTIAL DIAGNOSIS

Atypical varieties of measles, meningococcemia, drug eruptions, and even collagen vascular diseases can resemble Rocky Mountain spotted fever, but laboratory studies should differentiate these entities.

TREATMENT

Antimicrobial therapy is indicated with doxycycline, 100 mg bid, or tetracycline, 500 mg qid, for 5 to 7 days. Chloramphenicol may be used: 100 mg/kg IV up to 3 gm and then 50 mg/kg PO for 7 days. Sulfonamides are contraindicated.

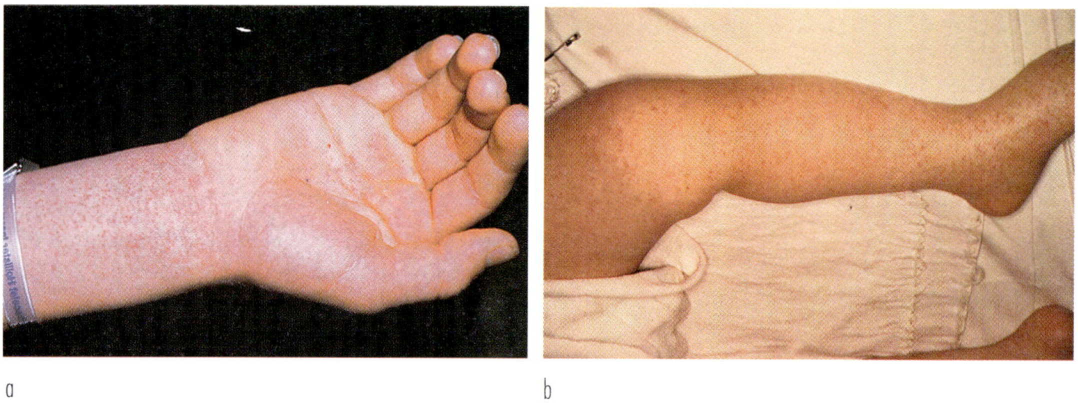

Figure 45
Rocky Mountain spotted fever may present as (a) fine erythematous macules. During the second week of the infection, (b) a petechial eruption may be found. (Courtesy of Susan Mallory, MD, St. Louis, MO.)

SUGGESTED READINGS

Dumler JS, Walker DH. Diagnostic tests for Rocky Mountain spotted fever and other rickettsial diseases. Dermatol Clin 1994; 12:25–36.

Kirk JL, Fine DP, Sexton DJ, et al. Rocky Mountain spotted fever: a clinical review base on 48 confirmed cases 1943-1986. Medicine 1990;69:35–45.

KIngston ME, Mackey D. Skin clues in the diagnosis of life-threatening infections. Rev Infect Dis 1986;8:1–11.

Sexton DJ, Corey GR: Rocky Mountain spotless and almost spotless fever: a wolf in sheep's clothing. Clin Infect Dis 1992; 15:439–448.

Spach DH, Liles WC, Campbell GL, et al. Tick-borne diseases in the United States. N Engl J Med 1993;329:935–947.

RICKETTSIALPOX

Rickettsialpox is a self-limiting disease with no fatalities reported.

ETIOLOGY

The causative agent is *Rickettsia akari*, an intracellular pathogen found in the house and field mouse, and is probably transmitted by *Lipnyssoides sanguineus*, a colorless mite. The disease has been found in New York and Philadelphia, as well as in parts of Russia, South Korea, and central Africa.

CLINICAL PRESENTATION

The disease is characterized by a triad of the initial eschar, fever, and a generalized erythematous macular to papular that leads to a vesicular eruption. The site of the mite bite is a red papule that becomes vesicular and then necrotic (Figure 46). Regional lymphadenopathy, fever, and an asymptomatic eruption develop over the next week on most parts of the body. By the second week, the lesions have cleared.

DIAGNOSIS

The diagnosis is made according to clinical suscipicion. Serologic confirmation is made by either complement fixation or immunofluorescence tests after the illness has been present for one week. The Weil-Felix reaction is negative.

DIFFERENTIAL DIANGOSIS

The eschar differentiates this rickettsial disease from other erythematous eruptions. The vesicular stage differs only from varicella, because all lesions are in the same stage of development.

TREATMENT

Therapy outlined for Rocky Mountain spotted fever is suggested.

SUGGESTED READINGS

Brettman LR, Lewin S, Halzman RS, et al. Rickettsialpox. Report of an outbreak and a contemporary review. Medicine 1991;60:363-372.

Burnett JW. Rickettsioses: a review for the dermatologist. J Am Acad Dermatol 1980;2:359-373.

Dumler JS, Walker DH. Diagnostic tests for Rocky Mountain spotted fever and other rickettsial diseases. Dermatol Clin 1994; 12:25-36.

Kass EM, Szaniawski WK, Levy H, et al. Rickettialpox in a New York City hospital, 1980–1989. N Engl J Med 1994;331:1612–1617.

Loubser MD, DAvies VA, Meyers KEC, et al. Severe illness cuased by *Rickettsia conorii*. Ann Trop Paediat 1993;13:277-280.

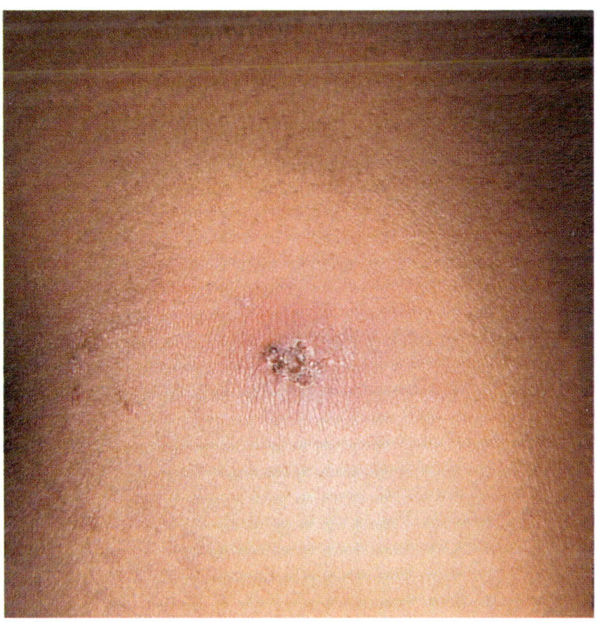

Figure 46
Rickettsialpox was the diagnosis made in this 56-year-old man as a result of the eschar. He had been admitted to the infectious disease service because of high fever.

Japanese Spotted Fever

Japanese spotted fever is one of the spotted fever diseases with specific geographic limitations.

ETIOLOGY

Rickettsia japonica has been identified as the pathogen, but the vector is unclear. *Amblyomma testdinarium, Haemaphysalis flava, H. longicornis,* and *Isodes ovatus* have been implicated, with the dog as the likely reservoir. Most cases have been reported from the southeast coast of Shikoku Island in bamboo bush workers and other agricultural laborers, particularly in the spring, summer, and fall.

CLINICAL PRESENTATION

Some 2 to 8 days following a suspected bite in the fields, an eschar forms at the site (Figure 47a). This is described as being a red indurated papule, 0.5 to 1.0 cm in diameter, with either a shallow ulcer or a central black crust (Figure 47b). There is also the abrupt onset of headache, remittent fever, and shaking chills. Within the next few days, an asymptomatic maculopapular eruption develops on the hands (including the palms), feet, and face, spreading quickly to cover most of the body (Figure 47c). The rash becomes petechial by the third or fourth day and disappears by the end of the second week, while the duration of the eschar ranges from 3 to 5 days, up to 14 days. Although there is no lymphadenopathy or enlargement of internal organs, hypotension and tachycardia are often found during the febrile period.

DIAGNOSIS

The Weil-Felix reaction (OX-2) becomes positive after the second week of the disease, whereas the OK-K and OK-19 are negative. The complement fixation test using *R. rickettsii* and *R. akari* are positive. The indirect immunoperoxidase test, utilizing Thai tick typhus and Katayama strain, is positive.

DIFFERENTIAL DIAGNOSIS

Japanese spotted fever resembles the typhus group of diseases. Scrub typhus has a larger eschar and no petechiae with generalized lymphadenopathy and hepatosplenomegaly.

TREATMENT

Tetracycline, 250 mg qid, or minocylcline, 100 mg bid, given for 14 days is recommended.

SUGGESTED READINGS

Boyd AS, Neldner KH. Typhus disease group. Int J Dermatol 1992;31:823-832.

McCalmont C, Zenolli MD. Rickettsial diseases. Dermatol Clin 1989;7:591-601.

Takada N, Fujita H, Yano Y, et al. Serosurveys of spotted fever and murine typhus in local residents of Taiwan and Thailand compared with Japan. Southeast Asian J Trop Med Public Health 1993;24:354-356.

Figure 47
The patient with Japanese spotted fever develops (a) an eschar, (b) an erythematous macular eruption, and (c) petechial lesions. (Courtesy of Fumihiko Mahara, MD, Anan City, Japan.)

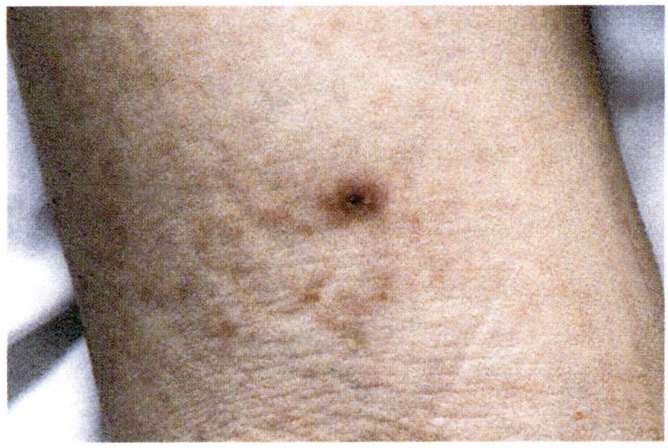

a

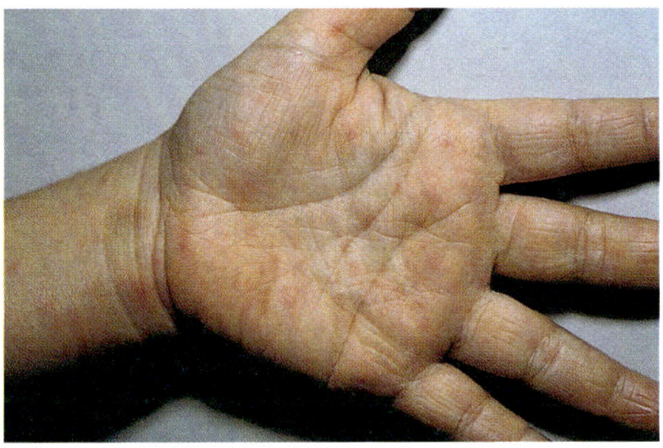

b

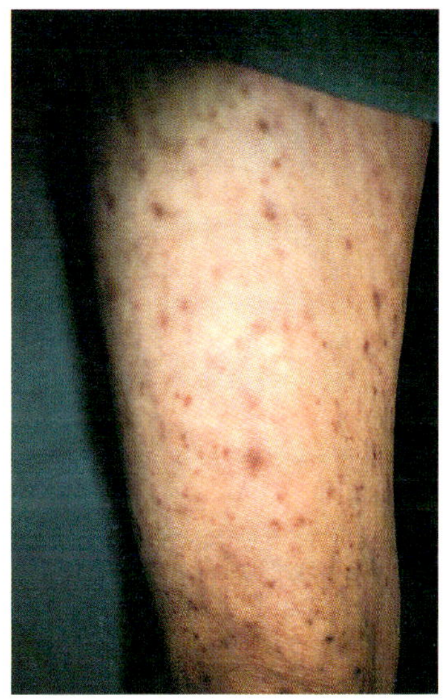

c

Boutonneuse Fever

Boutonneuse fever, also known as *Mediterranean fever, South African tick bite fever, Kenya tick typhus*, and *Indian tick typhus*, is notable for the initial lesion, an eschar.

ETIOLOGY

Rickettsia conorii is the causative agent and is found in field rodents and dogs. It is transmitted transovarially among ticks and indirectly by feeding on infected animals. The ixodid tick is the main vector. The disease is seen around the Mediterranean, Caspian, and Black sea basins, as well as in other parts of Africa, Pakistan, Thailand, and Malaysia.

CLINICAL PRESENTATION

A small painless red papule appears at thre sitre of the bite. The lesion soon ulcerates and forms a black eschar (tache noire) (Figure 48a). There may be multiple eschars in 10% of the patients. Sometimes, there is no visible eschar, but regional lymphadenopathy is common.

Systemic manifestations appear abruptly after a week-long incubation period. The severe headaches, malaise, and fever are followed in 3 to 5 days by an erythematous maculopapular (button-like) eruption appearing first on the extremities and rapidly spreading to the trunk (Figure 48b). The palms, soles, and face are involved. New crops of lesions continue to appear, until clearing beings in 7 to 10 days. Respiratory and gastrointestinal symptoms are common, and splenomegaly may occur.

DIAGNOSIS

R. conorii may be identified by an ELISA test. Histopathologic examination of the eschar shows a less severe lymphohistiocytic vasculitis and no thrombosis, as compared to Rocky Mountain spotted fever. Fluorescein-labeled (rabbit) globulin antiserum to *R. rickettsii* will identify *R. conorii* in the vessel walls.

DIFFERENTIAL DIAGNOSIS

This group of diseases resembles other ricksettsial diseases and may be differentiated by laboratory studies.

TREATMENT

Tetracycline, 250 mg qid, or ciprofloxacin, 500 mg bid, is effective. The antimicrobial is given until the eruption clears.

SUGGESTED READINGS

Boyd AS, Neldner KH. Typhus disease group. Int J Dermatol 1992;31:823–832.

Dujella J, Morovic M, Dzelalija B, Gveric M, et al. Histopatholpogy and immunopathology of skin biopsy specimens in Mediterranean spotted fever. Acta Virol (Praha) 1991;35:566–572.

Mansueto S, Tringali G, Walker DH. Widespread, simultaneous increase in the incidence of spotted fever group rickettsioses. J Infect Dis 1986; 154:539–540.

Figure 48
Boutonneuse fever is known by (a) the eschar that occurs at the site of the tick bite. (b) The eruption is characterized by an erythematous macular to papular eruption. (Courtesy of E. Joy Shultz, MD, Johanesburg, South Africa.)

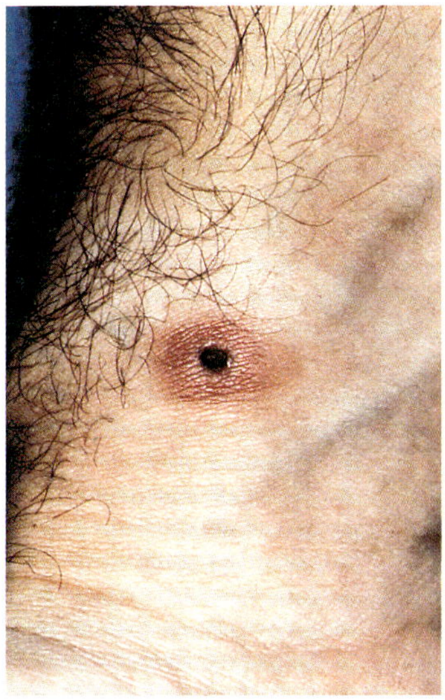

a

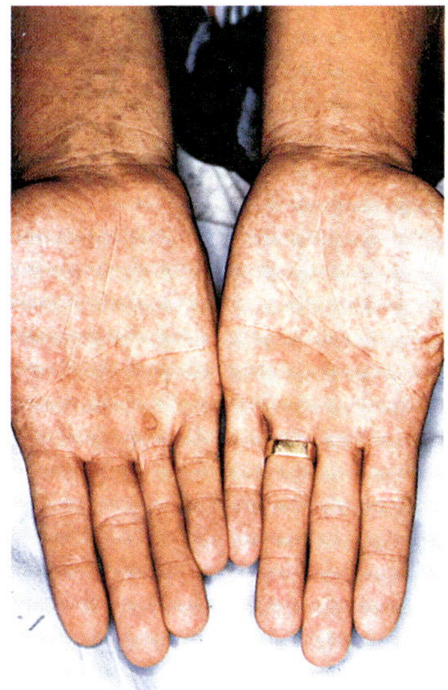

b

Loubser MD, Davies VA, Meyers KE, et al. Severe illness caused by Rickettsia conorii. Ann Trop Paediatr 1993;13:277–280.

Takada N, Fujita H, Yano Y, et al. Serosurveys oif spotted fever and murine typhus in local residents of Taiwan and Thailand compared with Japan. Southeast Asian J Med 1993;24:354–356.

Walker DH, Occhino C, Tringali GR, et al. Pathogenesis of rickettsial eschars: The tache noire of boutonneuse fever. Hum Pathol 1988;19:1449–1454.

Scrub Typhus

Scrub typhus (Tsutsugamushi fever) is an ancient disease found in the Orient from Korea to the northern part of Australia.

ETIOLOGY

Rickettsia tsutsugamushi has been recovered from rats, voles and field mice. Transmission to humans is through bites of chiggers, the larval form of the thzombiculid mites, usually *Leptotrobidium akamushi* or *L. deliensis*, which live in the grass, bush, or shrub-covered land. The incidence is highest in the summer and fall.

CLINICAL PRESENTATION

Within hours of chigger bites, small painless, red papules often appear. By the end of the first week, the lesions have become pustular, and they rupture to form ulcers, and finally, black eschars (Figure 49a).

Lymphadenopathy develops but may be confusing as not all patients have eschars. There is fever of 104°F or even 105°F with bradycardia. During the second week of the disease, the fever fluctuates and then subsides but constitutional symptoms of headache, cough, chills, malaise, and backache are common, as are conjunctival and pharyngeal hyperemia.

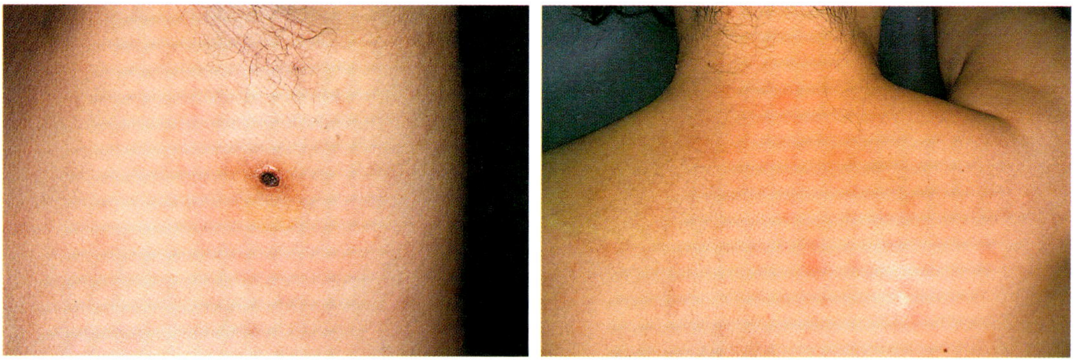

a b

Figure 49
Scrub typhus begins with (a) a black eschar surrounded by a zone of erythema, followed by (b) an erythematous macular eruption. (Courtesy of Yoshiki Taniguchi, MD, Tsu, Mie, Japan.)

An erythematous macular eruption without petechiae appears on the trunk during the fifth to eighth day of the fever. This rapidly becomes generalized and may involve the palms and soles (Figure 49b). The skin lesions last for 7 to 10 days. Without treatment, the mortality may reach 60% at the end of the second week due to pneumonitis, circulatory failure, renal failure, or encephalitis.

DIAGNOSIS

The polymerase chain reaction combined with microplate hybridization will prove the diagnosis within 6 hours. Immunoperoxidase and indirect fluorescent antibody tests also will confirm the diagnosis. The Weil-Felix test is also helpful with agglutination of the OX-K strain of Proteus found during convalescence. Histologic examination of the eruption will reveal vascultitis.

DIFFERENTIAL DIAGNOSIS

In endemic areas, the clinical presentation can be similar to other rickettsial diseases, malaria, viral exanthams, leptospirosis, and dengue fever. Laboratory studies are needed to differentiate the diseases.

TREATMENT

Tetracycline, 250 mg qid, for 14 days, is preferred over chloramphenicol, 50 mg/kg, although scrub typhus responds more rapidly than other rickettsial disease to therapy.

SUGGESTED READINGS

Boyd AS, Neldner KH. Typhus disease group. Int J Dermatol 1992;31:823–832.

Brown GW. Scrub typhus: pathogenesis and clinical syndrome. In: Walker DH, ed. Biology of rickettsial diseases, vol 1. Boca Raton, FL: CRC Press, 1988:93–100.

Currie B, O'Connor L, Dwyer B. A new focus of scrub typhus in tropical Australia. Am J Trop Med Hyg 1993;49:425–429.

Lee JS, Ahn C, Kim YK. Thirteen cases of rickettsial infection including nine cases of tsutsugamushi disease first confirmed in Korea. J Korean Med 1986;29:430–438.

Yi KS, Chong Y, Covington SC, et al. Scrub typhus in Korea: importance of early clinical diagnosis of this newly recognized endemic area. Mil Med 1993;158:269–273.

Bacillary Angiomatosis

Bacillary angiomatosis (BA); once called *epithelioid angiomatosis*, is a recently described cutaneous entity with systemic manifestations and is usually found in immunocompromised patients. It may be related to a zoonotic disease, bacillary peliosis.

ETIOLOGY

The causative organism is *Rochalimaea henselae* or *R. quintana*, a coccobacillus that is slightly gram-negative and appears to be similar to *Bartonella bacilliformis*, the agent of bartonellosis. It may also be the same agent of cat-scratch disease which was previously labeled *Afipia felis*. BA could be associated with injury to the skin by a cat.

CLINICAL PRESENTATION

There are three distinct types of BA: a pyogenic granulomatous form, a subcutaneous nodule (Figure 50), and a hyperpigmented indurated plaque form. The first are blood-red, smooth-surfaced papules. These somewhat tender lesions may be firm and friable, covered with crusted blood. The second are skin-colored or dusky subcutaneous nodules that may be tender. Sometimes, these nodules project above the skin. The third, which are usually found in African–American patients, are oval indurated plaques that may be purplish to hyperpigmented in color. Although the borders may be vague, the centers of the plaques may become hyperkeratotic.

In addition to cutaneous findings, there may be involvement of the bone, lymph nodes, spleen, liver, and soft tissue. A peculiar type of hepatic involvement characterized by blood-filled cysts known as peliosis hepatis occurs. Athough the lesions may even regress spontaneously, sometimes the growth of the internal lesions is so great that patients die of respiratory obstruction. BA may be accompanied by sweats, chills, weight loss, and weakness.

DIAGNOSIS

The clinical picture of BA is confirmed by histopathologic examination. There should be epithelial collarettes, lobular small-vessel proliferation, stromal edema, leukocytic infiltrates with leukocytoclastic debris, and purplish clumps of bacteria. With the Warthin-Starry stain, the tissue reveals brownish black bacilli in the perivascular areas. BA is also associated with bacillary peliosis

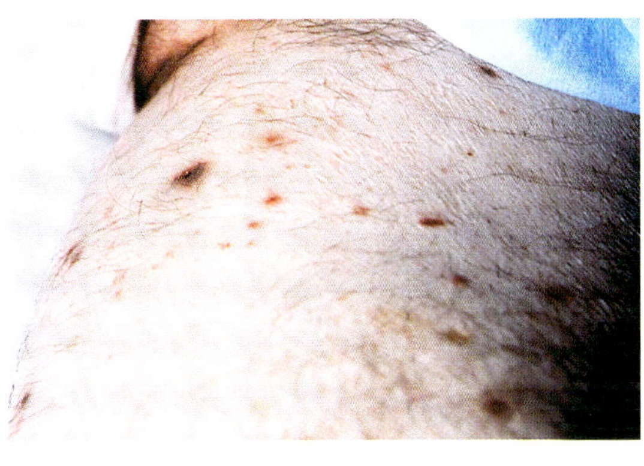

Figure 50
Bacillary angiomatosis presented as scattered red papules and nodules, some with crusting. (Courtesy of Burke Cunha, MD, Mineola, NY.)

DIFFERENTIAL DIAGNOSIS

BA may be confused with a number of benign lesions, ranging from pyogenic granuloma to verruca vulgaris and keratoacanthoma. Kaposi's sarcoma is a similar purplish nodule that can be distinguished by the evolution of the lesions and the histopathology.

TREATMENT

Macrolides, such as erythromycin (250–500 mg qid) or clarithryomycin (500 mg bid), administered for several weeks, are curative. Doxycycline,100 mg/day, and ciprofloxacin, 750 mg bid, are also useful antimicrobial agents in the treatment of BA. The penicillins and cephalosporins are not effective. Isolated lesions are amenable to curettage and electrodesiccation.

SUGGESTED READINGS

Cockerell CJ. The causative agent of bacillary angiomatosis. Int J Dermatol 1992;31:615–617.

Koehler JE, Tappero JW. Bacillary angiomatosis and bacillary peliosis in patients infected with human immunodeficiency virus. Clin Infect Dis 1993;17:12–24.

LeBoit PE. Bacillary angiomatosis: a systemic opportunistic infection with prominent cutaneous manifestations. Semin Dermatol 1991;10:194–198.

Spach DH. Bacillary angiomatosis. Int J Dermatol 1992;31:19–26.

Tappero J, Mohle-Boetani J, Koehler J, et al. The epidemiology of bacillary angiomatosis and bacillary peliosis. JAMA 1993;269:770–775.

Webster GF. Bacillary (epithelioid) angiomatosis. Clin Dermatol 1991;9:75–77.

Webster GF. The clinical spectrum of bacillary angiomatosis. Br J Dermatol 1992;126:535–541.

Cat-Scratch Disease

Cat-scratch disease (CSD), first described in 1950 and also called *benign lymphoreticulosis*, is characterized by vague cutaneous lesions, associated with inguinal or axillary lymphadenopathy. Seventy-five percent of the patients are children, who are most often afflicted from September to February.

ETIOLOGY

Afipia felis was believed to be the causative agent over the past decade; however, *Rochalimaea henselae*, a gram-negative coccobacillus, is now considered to be the bacterium involved. Transmission is by a cat bite or a scratch inflicted by a cat or thorn. Often, the cat may by infested with fleas.

CLINICAL PRESENTATION

One to 2 weeks following the injury, a papule, vesicle, or pustule may appear as the primary complex. This is often purplish and firm and ulceration is possible (Figure 51). Sometimes, a transient morbilliform eruption is present. Tender regional lymphadenopathy appears 1 to 4 weeks later and may suppurate. CSD usually clears within 6 weeks but may last up to 2 years. Malaise, fever, and weakness may accompany these findings. CSD is the leading cause of unilateral lymphadenopathy in patients in the first two decades of life.

The oculo-glandular syndrome of Parinaud is a variant of CSD. This represents a papule in the periorbital area, conjunctivitis, and associated periauricular lymphadenopathy. Erythema nodosum, erythema annulare, erythema marginatum, and purpura have also been reported in association with CSD.

DIAGNOSIS

The presence of cat scratches should suggest the diagnosis, which can be confirmed by biopsy. Staining the tissue with Warthin-Starry stain will reveal the clusters of gram-negative pleomorphic bacilli. Aspirating pus from an enlarged lymph node and staining with Warthin-Starry stain should also confirm the diagnosis. Previously, the Frei test was used, but this depends on obtaining pus from an infected patient. The Hanger and Rose skin test with cat-scratch antigen is positive 1 week after the appearance of adenitis.

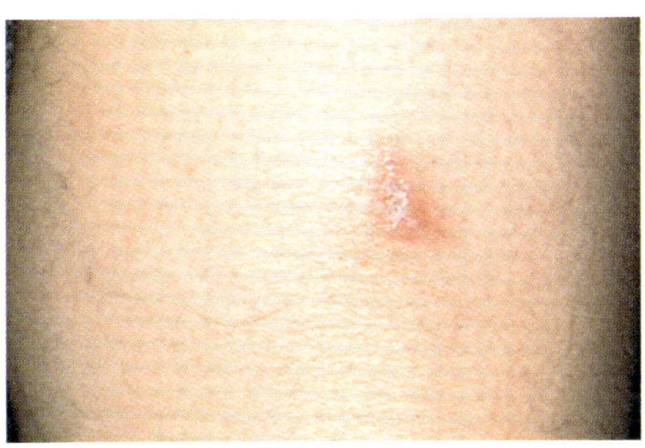

Figure 51
Cat-scratch disease developed a few days after a bite from the patient's pet cat. The area became red and nodular. (Courtesy of Roberto Arenas, MD, Mexico City, Mexico.)

DIFFERENTIAL DIAGNOSIS

Several infectious diseases, including sporotrichosis, atypical mycobacterial infection, cutaneous tuberculosis, and sarcoidosis may have suggestive presentations. Histological examination should then reveal the diagnosis.

TREATMENT

No treatment is needed in the normal host. If immunosuppression is suspected, erythromycin, 250 mg qid, or tetracycline, 250 mg qid, may be given for 10 to 14 days.

SUGGESTED READINGS

Dolan MJ, Wong MT, Regnery RL. Syndrome of *Rochalimea henselae* adenitis suggesting cat-scratch disease. Ann Intern Med 1993;118:331–336.

Gupta AK, Rasmussen JE. What's new in pediatric dermatology. J Am Acad Dermatol 1988;18:239–259.

Koehler JE, Glaser CA, Tappero JW. *Rochalimaea henselae* infection: a new zoonosis with the domestic cat as reservoir. JAMA 1994;271:531–535.

Margileth AM. Antibiotic therapy for cat-scratch disease: clinical study of therapeutic outcome in 268 patients and a review of the literature. Pediatr Infect Dis 1992;11:474–478.

Margileth AM, Hayden GF. Cat-scratch disease: from feline affection to human infection. N Engl J Med 1993;329:53–54.

Roberge RJ. Cat-scratch disease. Emerg Med Clin North Am 1991;9:327–334.

Shinall EA. Cat-scratch disease; a review of the literature. Pediatr Dermatol 1990; 7:11–18.

Tompkins DC, Steigbigel RT. *Rochalimaea's* role in cat scratch disease and bacillary angiomatosis. Ann Intern Med 1993;118:388–389.

Bartonellosis

Bartonellosis represents Oroya fever and verruca peruana. It is sometimes called Carrion's disease, after Daniel Carrion, the medical student who died investigating the disease.

ETIOLOGY

The causative agent is *Bartonella bacilliformis*, a gram-negative coccobacillus, closely related to the causative agents of bacillary angiomatosis and cat-scratch disease. The organism may have a reservoir in some animals, with dogs and rats known to have latent infections.

The bacillus is transmitted by the *Phlebotomus* fly, although in Colombia ticks and lice have been implicated. Following a bite, the incubation period for the disease to become full-blown ranges from 2 weeks to 4 months.

CLINICAL PRESENTATION

There are two phases of the infection, both of which are found in South America, particularly in Peru, Bolivia, Colombia, and Ecuador.

Oroya fever (OF), the hematinic phase, is characterized by hemolytic anemia, arthralgia, and myalgia. Lymphadenopathy, hepatosplenomegaly, and jaundice may occur. The fever lasts for 1 to 3 weeks and has no skin lesions other than the initial insect bite at the site of inoculation, but it can be severe enough to be fatal. Most patients who recover from the febrile stage of OF will develop verruca peruana (VP).

The histoid phase of VP has multiple cherry-red, hard, verrucous lesions of varying size on the skin and mucous membranes. Although the lesions are painless, there may be underlying joint pain and fever. Nodular lesions develop in the subcutaneous tissue over the elbows and knees. Gradually, they can become ulcerated and hemorrhagic. After 2 to 12 weeks, the tumors may resorb, sometimes leaving scars. Secondary infection with salmonella is a major problem, but VP is generally benign (Figure 52a,b).

DIAGNOSIS

In OF, examination of a blood smear stained with Giemsa would show the bacteria in the erythrocytes. In VP, skin biopsy would reveal the gram-negative organisms in the edematous endothelial cells. Histologically, there are proliferating angioblastic cells and an inflammatory infiltrate of plasma cells and leukocytes. The proliferating vessels and endothelial cells often suggest capillary hemangiomas.

DIFFERENTIAL DIAGNOSIS

The skin lesions may be confused with pyogenic granulomas, ulcerated hemangiomas, or Kaposi's sarcoma.

TREATMENT

While OF can be treated with penicillin, tetracycline, and chloramphenicol, VP requires chloramphenicol, 2 to 3 gm/day for 8 days.

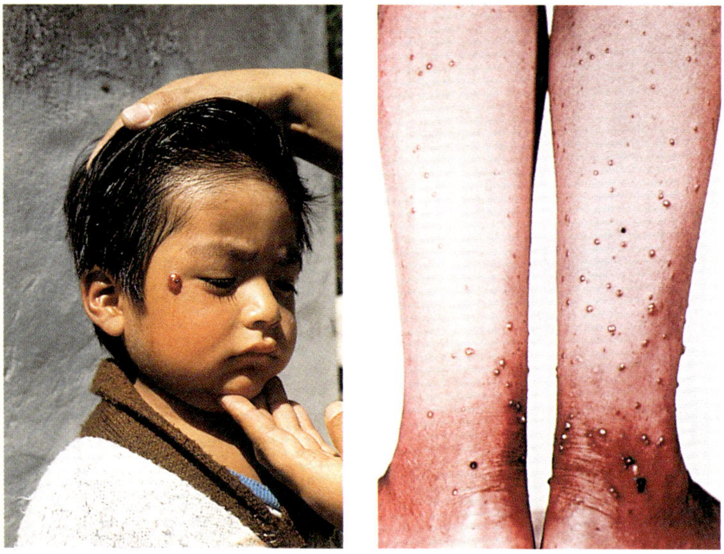

Figure 52
Bartonellosis appeared in this boy as (a) a purplish nodule on the temple. (Courtesy of JE Arrese, MD and GE Pierard, MD, Liege, Belgium. Reproduced with permission from Piel 1992;7:49.) (b) Sometimes, it is widespread, with distinct verrucous lesions; hence the appellation of verruca peruviana.

SUGGESTED READINGS

Garcia FU, Wojta J, Broadley KN, et al. *Bartonella bacilliformis* stimulates endothelial cells in vitro and is angiogenic in vivo. Am J Pathol 1990;136:1125–1135.

Garcia-Caceres U, Garcia FU. Bartonellosis. An immunodepressive disease and the life of Daniel Alcides Carrion. Am J Clin Pathol 1991; 95(suppl 1):S58–S66.

Leonard J. Daniel Carrión and Carrión's disease. Bull Can Am Healthg Organ 1991;25:258–266.

Ricketts WE. Clinical manifestations of Carrion's disease. Arch Inter Med 1949; 84:751–781.

CHLAMYDIAE

Chlamydiae are obligate intracellular gram-negative bacteria. They are larger than viruses, being 300 to 500 nm in diameter. Unlike viruses, they contain both DNA and RNA. Unlike other bacteria, they have two morphologic states—extracellular and intracellular. The basophilic intracytoplasmic inclusion bodies are shown by Castaneda stain.

CHLAMYDIAL INFECTIONS

Chlamydial infections include psittacosis and a pneumonia. *Chlamydia trachomatis* is responsible for one of the most common sexually transmitted diseases, a nonspecific urethritis, and trachoma.

LYMPHOGRANULOMA VENEREUM

Lymphogranuloma venereum is a sexually transmitted disease that is predominantly found in the tropics.

ETIOLOGY

C. trachomatis, immunotypes L_1, L_2, and L_3, causes this affliction of the lymphatic channels.

CLINICAL PRESENTATION

The initial papule, which is rarely found, develops on the sexual contact area within days or weeks of exposure. Ten to 30 days later, the solitary lesion usually ulcerates and presents a chancreform picture. Then, an inguinal syndrome, comprised of femoral, usually unilateral, inguinal, and perirectal lymphadenopathy, develops. These nodes become swollen and fluctuant. Because of the pressure exerted above and below Poupart's ligament, the buboes create an indentation or groove sign (Figure 53a). They may also ulcerate. Other complications include perirectal abscesses and ischiorectal and rectovaginal fistulas. There is elephantiasis of the vulva, with ulceration called *esthiomene* (Figure 53b), and there may be associated arthritis and erythema nodosum.

DIAGNOSIS

The chlamydial complement fixation test is the most reliable. There are antigen detection tests using direct immunofluorescence (DIF) and enzymes (enzyme immunoassay, EIA), which are rapid, fairly specific, and equally sensitive. Previously, the Frei test was used but it proved to be too nonspecific. Smears of pus are very unreliable.

DIFFERENTIAL DIAGNOSIS

This condition may initially be confused with herpes progenitalis owing to the group of papules, while the ulceration can mimic syphilis and chancroid.

TREATMENT

Doxycycline, 100 mg bid, or tetracycline, 500 qid, for 21 days is effective. Erythromycin, 500 mg qid for 21 days, can also be used.

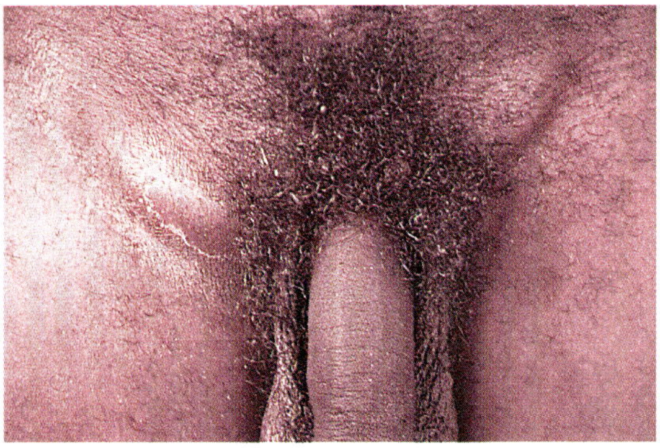

a

Figure 53
(a) Charcteristic of lymphogranuloma venereum are the groove sign and bubo. (b) In esthiomene, there is marked swelling of the vulva.

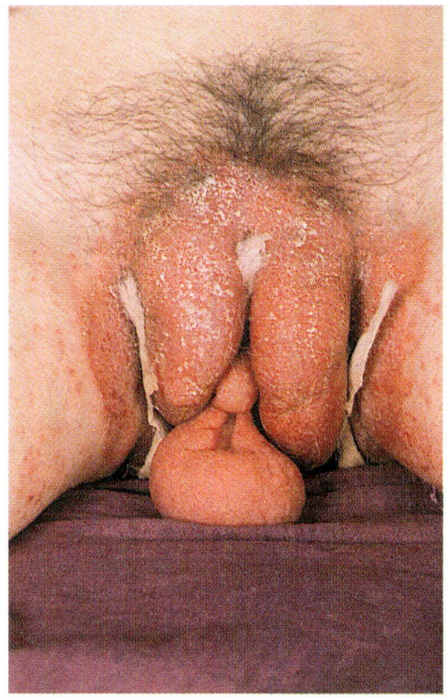

b

SUGGESTED READINGS

Allegra F. Lymphogranuloma venereum. In: Parish LC, Gschnait F. Sexually transmitted diseases: a guide for clinicians. New York: Springer-Verlag, 1989:90–104.

Elgart ML. Sexually transmitted diseases of the vulva. Dermatol Clin 1992;10:387–403.

Mroczkowski TF, Martin DH. Genital ulcer disease. Dermatol Clin 1994;12:753–764.

Goh BT, Forster GE. Sexually transmitted diseases in children: chlamydial oculogenital infection. Genitourin Med 1993;69:213–221.

Mroczkowski TF, Martin DH. Genital ulcer disease. Dermatol Clin 1994;12:753–764.

Oehme A, Musholt PB, Dreesbach K. Chlamydiae as pathogens—an overview of diagnostic techniques, clinical features, and therapy of infections. Klin Wochenschr 1991;69:463–473.

Parish LC, Seghal VN, Buntin DM. Color atlas of sexually transmitted diseases. New York: Igaku-Shoin, 1991:112–117.

Rubinstein N, Granat M, Kopolovic Y, et al. Esthiomene: report of a case in a young Israeli woman. Int J Dermatol 1983;22:534–535.

Schacter J, Osoba HO. Lymphogranuloma venereum. Br Med Bull 1983;39:151–154.

Van Dyck E, Piot P. Laboratory techniques in the investigation of chancroid, lymphograuloma venereum and donovanosis. Genitourin Med 1992;68:130–133.

VIRUSES

Viruses are small enough that they cannot be visualized under the light microscope. These organisms that live and reproduce within living cells are antigenic and frequently mutate. All viruses contain nucleic acid and can be categorized according to their DNA or RNA content.

VIRAL INFECTIONS

The vast majority of viral infections may have no cutaneous signs. Many virally induced diseases are characterized by a prodromal phase of malaise, fever, and headache, whereas other viral diseases may have localized inflammation.

FARMYARD-POX

Milker's nodules and orf, also known as *ecthyma contagiosum* and *ecthyma infectiosum*, are two zoonotic diseases so similar in scope that they might be grouped together as farmyard-pox.

ETIOLOGY

These zoonoses are caused by parapoxviruses whose characteristics can only be distinguished by tissue culture. They cause udderpox or falsepox in cattle and lip scab in sheep. The virus is transmitted to humans by contact with contaminated animals or objects, something that occurs easily among animal handlers, as the virus is resistant to heat, cold, and drying.

CLINICAL PRESENTATION

Both milker's nodules and orf are characterized by single or multiple inflamed nodular lesions, 1 to 3 cm in diameter, that appear at the site of infection. Following an incubation period of a few days up to 11 days, a cherry-red papule appears (Figure 54a). The surrounding area becomes erythematous and indurated before the central part becomes purpuric and then necrotic (Figure 54b). Secondary bacterial infection can occur, prior to resolution in 4 to 6 weeks.

DIAGNOSIS

Electron microscopy will reveal the virions, and tissue culture techniques can be used to confirm the diagnosis. Pox virus replicates in cytoplasm. If the patient was exposed to cattle, the diagnosis of milker's nodules could be made. If the patient was in contact with sheep, then orf is the diagnosis. Histopathologically, there are viral inclusion bodies, capillary proliferation, and pseudoepitheliomatous hyperplasia.

DIFFERENTIAL DIAGNOSIS

Histopathologic study will differentiate a keratoacanthoma and a pyogenic granuloma. Microbiologic studies will distinguish tuberculosis verrucosa cutis.

TREATMENT

Symptomatic treatment with saline or Burow's 1:40 solution compresses may be used.

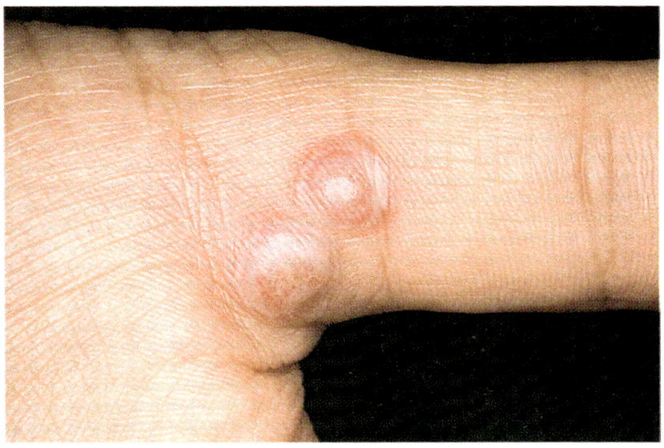

a

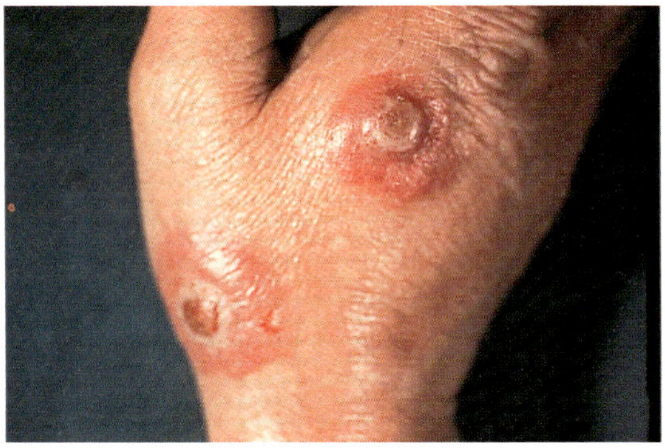

b

Figure 54
Orf begins as (a) red papulovesicular lesions with early central necrosis that over several days (b) become frankly necrotic. (Courtesy of Guy Chabeau, MD Lyon, France.)

SUGGESTED READINGS

Groves R, Wilson-Jones E, MacDonald DM. Human orf and milker's nodule: a clinicopathologic study. J Am Acad Dermatol 1991;25:706–711.

Johannessen JV, Krogh H-K, Solberg I. Human orf. J Cutan Pathol 1975;2:265–283.

Nagington J, Tee GH, Smith JG. Milker's nodule virus infections in Dorset and their similarity to orf. Nature 1965;208:505–507.

Shelley WB, Shelley ED. Farmyard pox: parapox virus infection in man. Br J Dermatol 1983;108:725–727.

Yirrell DL, Vestey JP, Norval M. Immune responses of patients to orf virus infection. Br J Dermatol 1994;130:438–443.

Molluscum Contagiosum

Molluscum contagiosum is a common skin disease that once was believed to be limited to children but is now found in all age groups.

ETIOLOGY

Molluscum contagiosum is caused by a large DNA virus of the pox family. Two types are currently known. Transmission is by personal contact.

CLINICAL PRESENTATION

The characteristic lesions are 1 to 5 mm in diameter, dome-shaped, skin-colored to pearly white papules, frequently with umbilicated centers. They are found on most parts of the body, except for the palms and soles, and generally spontaneously disappear within a year (Figure 55a). Rarely, they are found in the mouth or the conjunctiva (Figure 55b). Children are frequently afflicted, but the lesions can also be seen in adults, often in those with sexually transmitted or immunologic diseases.

DIAGNOSIS

The clinical picture can be confirmed by nicking the surface of the lesion. The globules that are exposed then can be smeared on a slide and stained with Wright or gram solution to show cytoplasmic inclusion bodies.

DIFFERENTIAL DIAGNOSIS

The lesions are usually recognized with ease, but sometimes they can be confused with warts. Large lesions may even resemble epithelial cysts. Similar lesions may be caused by cryptococcosis or histoplasmosis in patients with the human immunodeficiency virus (HIV).

TREATMENT

If the patient wishes to have the lesions removed, they can be easily nicked with a scissors or scalpel and the contents expressed. Keratolytic agents, such as a 6% salicylic acid gel, can be used to peel down the lesions, or cantharidin-containing compounds may be applied to the lesions to blister them.

SUGGESTED READINGS

Epstein WL. Molluscum contagiosum. Semin Dermatol 1992;11:184–189.

Ghigliotti G, Carrega G, Farris A, et al. Cutaneous cryptococcosis resembling molluscum contagiosum in a homosexual man with AIDS. Acta Derm Venereol (Stockh) 1992;72:182–184.

Gottlieb SL, Myskowski PL. Molluscum contagiosum. Int J Dermatol 1994;33:453–461.

Williams LR, Webster GW. Warts and molluscum contagiosum. Clin Dermatol 1991;9:87–93.

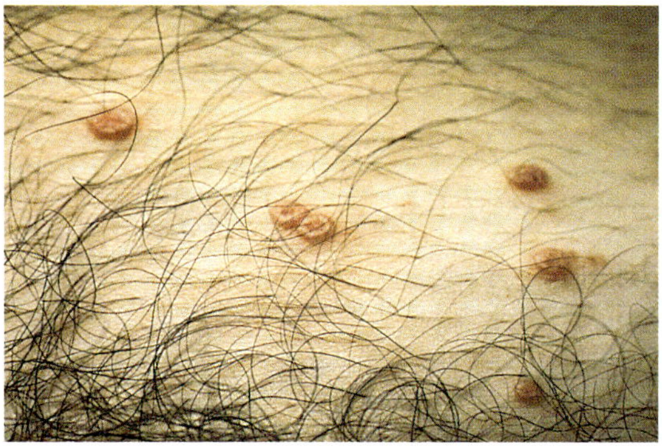

a

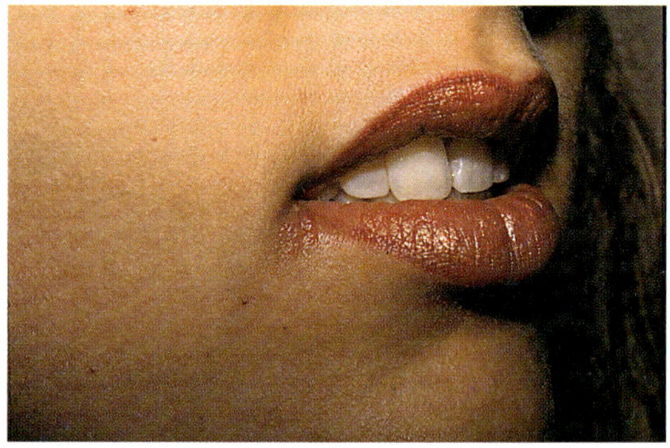

b

Figure 55
(a) Molluscum contagiosum presents as umbilicated reddish papules. (b) Sometimes this viral infection can be deceiving, when it is present at the oral commissure.

VERRUCAE

Verrucae represent a collection of diseases ranging from common warts to condyloma acuminata and from laryngeal papilloma to epidermodysplasia verruciformis of Lewandowsky.

ETIOLOGY

This human papillomavirus (HPV) currently is known to have more than 70 types. It is a member of the papovavirus group and has double-stranded DNA. Once the virus is introduced into the skin, it seems to remain for many years.

CLINICAL PRESENTATION

Warts may range from 1 mm, barely perceptible, flat lesions to 2- to 3-cm, elevated, hyperkeratotic lesions with reddish brown dots. They are generally asymptomatic but can create pruritus and tenderness (Figure 56a,b).

DIAGNOSIS

Although the clinical manifestations usually are self-evident, occasionally a biopsy will be needed to confirm the diagnosis. In genital warts, dilute acetic acid applied to the warts may highlight the lesions.

DIFFERENTIAL DIAGNOSIS

Infrequently, the wart may be confused with a molluscum contagiosum, seborrheic keratosis, or stucco keratosis, but the reddish brown dots are pathognomonic for warts. Surgical excision often leads to recurrence plus a painful scar.

TREATMENT

No treatment is more than 70% effective. New warts can rapidly appear at the treatment site. Cryosurgery, electrosurgery, laser surgery, radiotherapy, surgical excision, or chemosurgery each has its own merits and deficiencies.

SUGGESTED READINGS

Egawa K. New types of human papillomaviruses and intracytoplasmic inclusion bodies: a classification of inclusion warts according to clinical features, histology and associated HPV types. Br J Dermatol 1994;130:158–166.

Jablonska S, Orth G. Warts/human papillomaviruses. Clin Dermatol 1985;3(4):1–220.

Kling AR. Genital warts-therapy. Semin Dermatol 1992;11:247–255.

Ling MR. Therapy of genital human papillomavirus infections. I: Indications for and justification of therapy. Int J Dermatol 1992;31:682–686.

Ling MR. Therapy of genital human papillomavirus infections. II: Methods of treatment. Int J Dermatol 1992;31:769–776.

Monsonego J. Medical treatments of papillomavirus lesions: realities and future. Nouv Dermatol 1994;13:3–11.

Williams LR, Webster GW. Warts and molluscum contagiosum. Clin Dermatol 1991;9:87–93.

Figure 56
Verrucae may present (a) with a typical warty digitate picture as shown on this man's face or (b) as confluent warty overgrowths (condyloma acuminatum) on the penis of an HIV-positive patient.

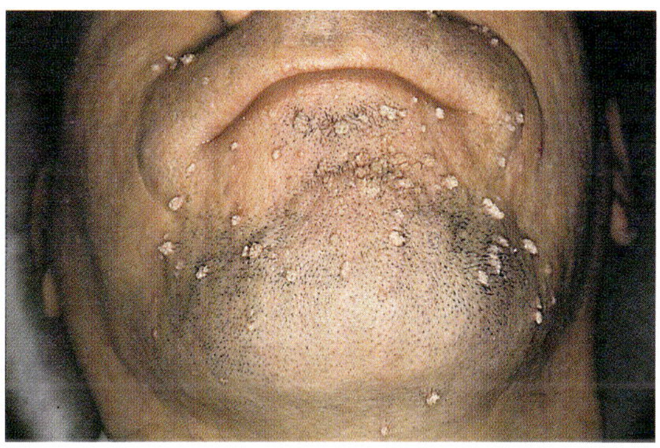

a

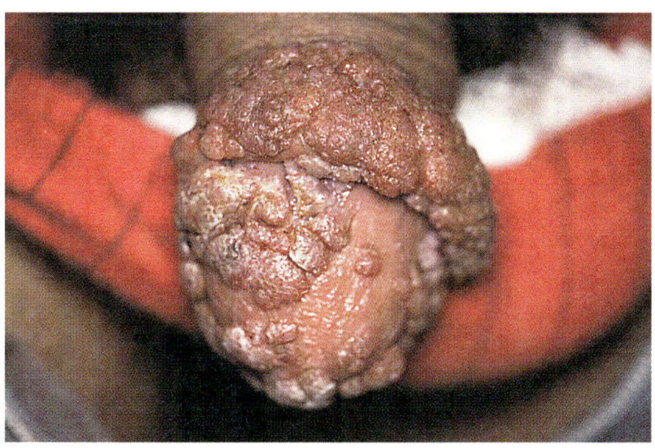

b

Herpes Simplex Virus Infection

Herpes simplex virus (HSV) infection has a variety of names reflecting location: *herpes simplex labialis* (cold sore or fever blister) and *herpes progenitalis* (genital herpes) (see Table 7).

ETIOLOGY

HSV is a karyotypic DNA virus that is classified into types 1 and 2. Type 1 is found predominantly above the waistline and type 2 in the genitalia, but neither location is mutually exclusive. The virus has a propensity for nerve tissue and hence lives in the dorsal root ganglia. Over 90% of the population has had HSV infection at any one time, and most are aymptomatic.

Table 7 Types of the Human Herpesvirus

Type	Associated disease
HHV-1, HSV-1	herpes simplex infection, type 1
HHV-2, HSV-2	herpes simplex infection, type 2
HHV-3, VZV	varicella, herpes zoster infection
HHV-4, EBV	infectious mononucleosis (Epstein-Barr virus disease)
HHV-5, HCMV	human cytomegalovirus disease
HHV-6	exanthe subitum (sixth disease)

CLINICAL PRESENTATION

Within 2 to 20 days following contact with the virus, the primary infection may occur (Figure 57a). This is characterized by red papules that become tense vesicles, often with crusting and purulence. The area is tender and sore with regional lymphadenopathy. Fever and malaise may accompany the primary eruption which can occur on any part of the body (i.e., finger—herpetic whitlow or paronychia; eczematized skin—Kaposi's varicelliform eruption; female genitalia—vulvovaginitis herpetica; and mouth—gingivostomatitis).

The primary eruption subsides and the virus retreats to the dorsal root ganglia. Recurrences then occur at the primary site, triggered by sunburn, fever, trauma, or unknown causes. The characteristic herpetic lesion then develops with grouped vesicles or vesiculopustular lesions, surrounded by erythema and sometimes induration. There may be prodromal symptoms of itching, fever, and malaise. Intervals between attacks may range from a few weeks to several years. Often, the virus never surfaces again. The recurrent form of HSV infection may be named according to location, such as those of the mouth (herpes labialis) (Figure 57b) and genitalia (herpes progenitalis) (Figure 57c). The buttocks (Figure 57d) may become infected, but patients rarely are aware of this location.

Infection with HSV is recognized as a cause of erythema multiforme. The latter may be preceded only by the prodrome or by a regular outbreak of a cold sore or genital herpes. In immunosuppressed patients, there is a chronic progressive ulcerative form of HSV infection.

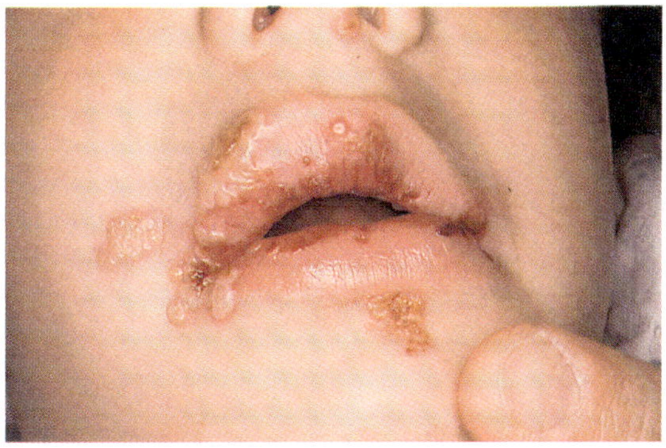

a

Figure 57
(a) Herpes simplex infection first appears as a primary eruption with tense, painful vesicles and pustules at the site of inoculation. (b) Recurrent attacks on the lips, known as herpes labialis, are often due to type 1 HSV infection. (c) Lesions on the genitalia, herpes progenitalis, are frequently due to type 2 HSV infection. In this patient, the recurrent lesions were on the mouth, whereas those on the genitalia were present for the first time. (d) Another site of infection may be the buttocks.

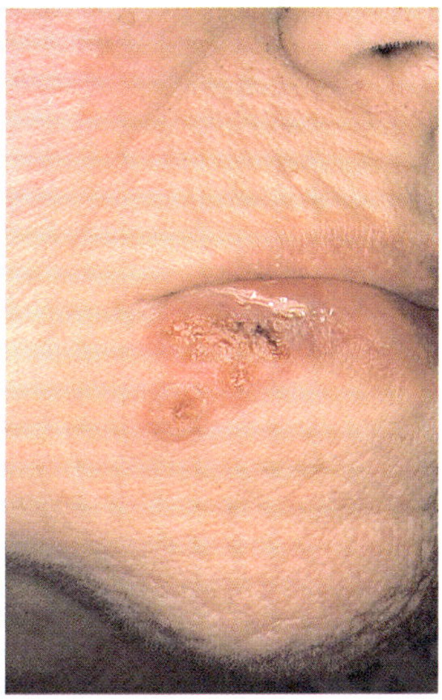

b

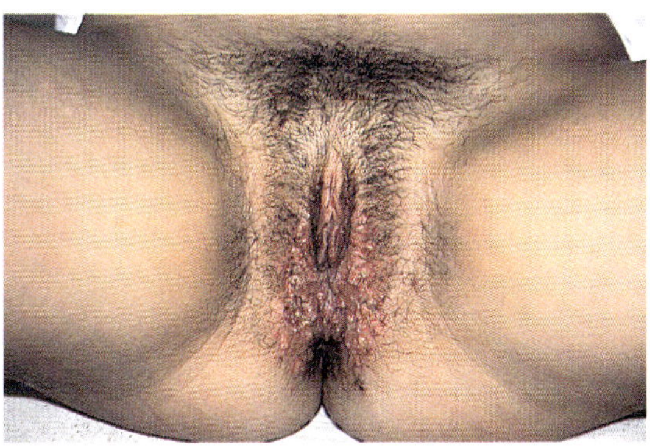

c

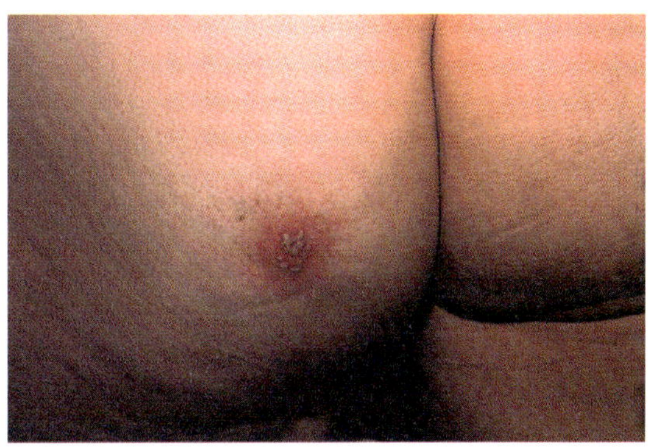

d

DIAGNOSIS

The clinical suspicion can be substantiated by a positive viral culture, which is more accurate than a Tzanck smear in herpes simplex infection. For the latter, the material from the base of a vesicle is smeared on a glass slide and is stained with hematoxylin-eosin, Giemsa, or Papanicolaou. Multinucleate giant epidermal cells are also seen on histopathologic examination of a biopsy specimen. Complement fixation serologic tests may also be helpful. Seroconversion occurs following a primary infection; if the result is negative, then HSV can be ruled out.

DIFFERENTIAL DIAGNOSIS

A herpes simplex infection can be confused with contact dermatitis, impetiga, or insect bites, but the recurrent nature of the infection and the laboratory tests will reveal the diagnosis.

TREATMENT

Acyclovir, 200 mg PO 5 times a day for 10 to 14 days, given during the prodromal phase or at the onset of the cutaneous lesions will abort the attack. Recurrent attacks may be prevented with indefinite use of acyclovir, 200 mg bid or tid. Symptomatic relief can be obtained by using Burow's 1:40 solution compresses tid and topical steroids.

SUGGESTED READINGS

Chang T-W. Herpes Simplex Virus. Clin Dermatol 1984;2(2):1–156.

Huff JC. Erythema multiforme and latent herpes simplex infection. Semin Dermatol 1992;11:207–210.

Solomon AR, Rasmussen JE, Varani J, et al. The Tzanck smear in the diagnosis of cutaneous herpes simplex. JAMA 1984;251:633–635.

Spruance SL. The natural history of recurrent oral-facial herpes simplex virus infection. Semin Dermatol 1992;11:200–206.

Vanderhooft S, Kirby P. Genital herpes simplex virus infection: natural history. Semin Dermatol 1992;11:190–199.

Varicella-Zoster Virus

Varicella (chickenpox) and herpes zoster infection (shingles) are the result of the same herpesvirus.

ETIOLOGY

The varicella-zoster virus (VZV) is herpesvirus 3, which consists of double-stranded DNA. The virus apparently remains in the dorsal root ganglia after the childhood disease and surfaces later in life to cause herpes zoster infection.

CLINICAL PRESENTATION

Chickenpox begins 4 to 6 days following contact, with the initial site of infection being the conjunctiva or the upper respiratory tract mucosa. Following a viremia, the virus invades the epidermis, producing macules, papules, and then vesicles. The lesions usually develop on the trunk and face before spreading to the extremities. New vesicles then appear in crops over the next few days, and old lesions become pustular and crusted. As a result, there are three different types of lesions on the body during the 3- to 5-day period. The patient may have malaise and fever. The lesions are pruritic and sometimes heal with depressed scars (Figure 58a,b). Oral lesions are composed of whitish erosions and vesicles (Figure 58c).

Herpes zoster infection starts with vague symptomatology. There is itching or discomfort along a dermatome. After several days, vesicles surrounded by redness appear in groups. The lesions may become pustular, resulting in confluent crusting. The disease often resolves within a month but not without leaving pain and scarring in some patients, the former being more severe in older patients. When the infection involves the geniculate ganglion, the disease is known as the *Ramsay Hunt syndrome* (Figure 58d,e).

DIAGNOSIS

The clinical picture is confirmed by a Tzanck smear, whereby the contents of the base of a vesicle are smeared on a slide. Multinucleate giant epidermal cells or nuclear inclusion bodies are seen. Viral cultures, which are less accurate in diagnosing these diseases than the Tzanck smear, and complement fixation tests are, nevertheless, helpful.

DIFFERENTIAL DIAGNOSIS

When smallpox still existed, it was distinguished from chickenpox as the former had umbilicated pustules and the lesions began on the extremities (Figure 58f). Other viral diseases may look similar at first, but the differentiation occurs as the disease progresses. Rarely, scabies or insect bites might be confused with chickenpox.

Herpes zoster infection is most distinctive because it occurs only on one side of the body, except in immunocompromised patients. An echovirus infection, impetigo, or insect bites might be confused if the lesions are localized.

Differentiating herpes zoster infection in an adult from primary HSV infection or the latter from the former in a child is difficult. Chickenpox is less severe and generally not localized. Localized HSV infection may also be very difficult to distinguish, but it usually is recurrent, unlike chickenpox.

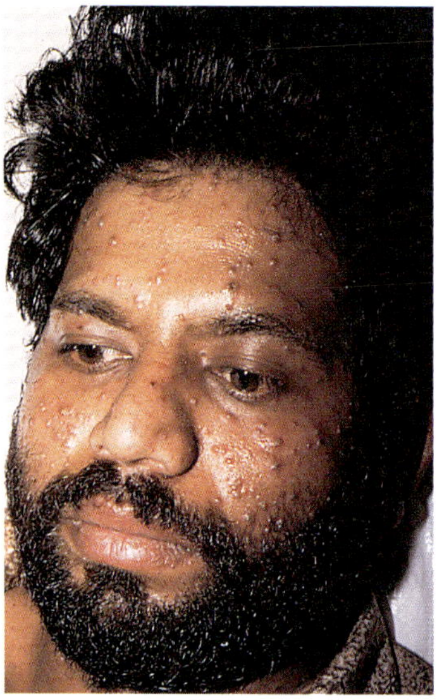

a

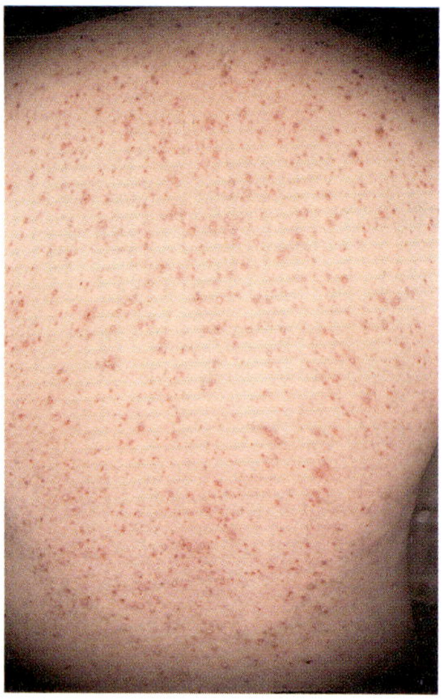

b

Figure 58
(a) Varicella is characterized by lesions in three stages: vesicles, pustules, and crusts. (b) Occasionally, papules predominate in the affected areas. (c) Oral lesions sometimes accompany chickenpox. (Courtesy of Charles Barr, DDS, New York, NY.) (d) Herpes zoster infection appears along the distribution of the affected nerve. This elderly man had herpes zoster ophthalmicus. (e) The segmental distribution of herpes zoster infection is shown on this patient. (f) Although smallpox is probably extinct, the clinical picture is characterized by umbilicated pustules that covered this Indian patient's face. All lesions are in the same stage, with greater involvement of the face, hands, and feet. (Courtesy of Günter Stüttgen, MD, Berlin, Germany.)

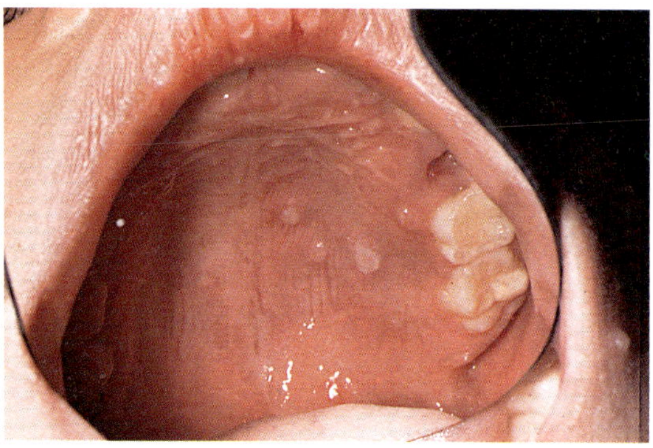

c

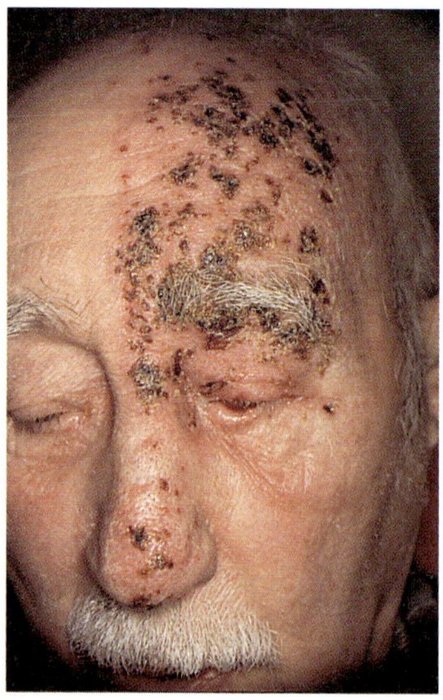

d

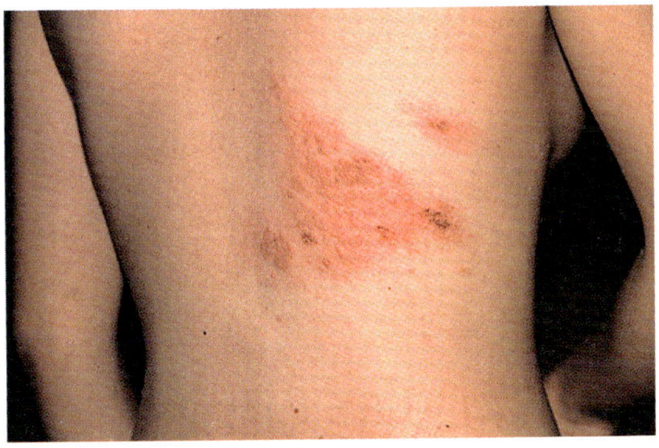

e

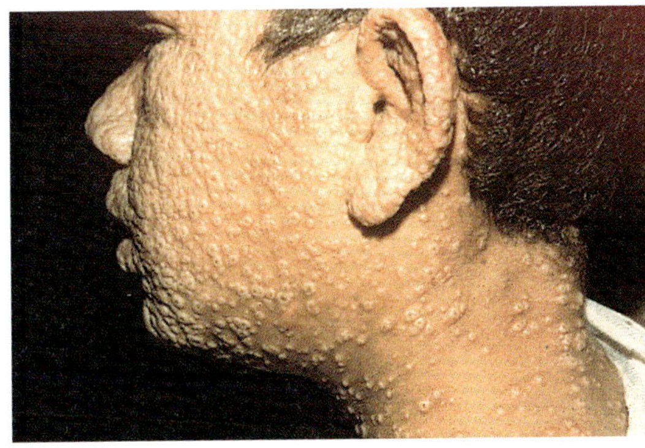

f

TREATMENT

Both diseases can be ameliorated if therapy with acyclovir or famciclovir is begun in the prodromal stage or just when the cutaneous lesions appear. The recommended dosage for acyclovir is 800 mg PO five times a day for 10 to 14 days or 500 mg PO tid for famciclovir. Symptomatic therapy for both diseases involves colloidal baths, twice daily, for 20 minutes, and topical steroids.

The itching of chickenpox may require antihistamines, such as hydroxyzine: children under 6 years, 50 mg PO, in divided doses; children over 6 years, 50 to 100 mg PO, in divided doses; and adults, 25 to 50 mg PO q6–8h. The pain of zoster often requires increasingly more powerful analgesics. Topical capsaicin, applied at least four times daily, is helpful.

SUGGESTED READINGS

Arvin AM. Cell-mediated immunity to varicella-zoster virus. J Infect Dis 1992; 166(suppl 1): S35–S41.

Cohen PR. Tests for detecting herpes simplex virus and varicella-zoster virus infections. Dermatol Clin 1994;12:51–68.

Gilden DH. Herpes zoster with postherpetic neuralgia—persisting pain and frustration. N Engl J Med 1994;330:932–933.

Liesegang TJ. The varicella-zoster virus: systemic and ocular features. J Am Acad Dermatol 1984;11:165–191.

Rockley PF, Tyring SK. Pathophysiology and clinical manifestations of varicella zoster virus infections. Int J Dermatol 1994;33:227–232.

Rowbotham MC. Treatment of postherpetic neuralgia. Semin Dermatol 1992;11:218–225.

Solomon AR, Rasmussen JE, Weiss JS. A comparison of the Tzanck smear and viral isolation in varicella and herpes zoster. Arch Dermatol 1986;122:282–285.

Tyring SK. Natural history of varicella zoster virus. Semin Dermatol 1992;11:211–217.

Enteroviral Exanthems

Enteroviral exanthems represent those eruptions due to such viruses as the coxsackie virus and echovirus groups. Most of the dermatologic findings are vague and nonspecific, but a few of the enteroviral exanthems are distinctive enough to be identified as separate entities.

ETIOLOGY

The enteroviruses are classified as RNA viruses, of which there are 160 types. These picornaviruses include polio and hepatitis A, as well as coxsackieviruses, echoviruses, and the intermediate enteroviruses.

CLINICAL PRESENTATION

Herpangina is due to coxsackievirus type A, types 1 through 10, 16, and 25, or echovirus types 3, 6, 9, 16, 17, 25, and 30. It often occurs in the summer in children. Following a 2- to 9-day incubation period, there is an abrupt onset of fever, malaise, and headache. Soon, pharyngitis and dysphagia appear, after which the small vesicles with red areolae appear on the pharynx and mucous membranes. They quickly evolve into grayish yellow ulcers that may necrose and ulcerate. Although the fever abates in 4 days, the pharyngeal redness and the exanthem take a few more days to disappear (Figure 59).

Hand, foot, and mouth disease is caused by coxsackievirus A16 and sometimes 4, 5, 7, 9, and 10, B 2 and 5, with an occasional outbreak due to enterovirus 71. Young children first develop a fever and sore throat after an incubation period of 3 to 5 days. The throat becomes red, and vesicles appear on pharynx, tongue, and gums (Figure 60a). Accompanying this exanthem are herpetic lesions that are vesicles surrounded by erythema on the ventral surface of the hands and feet (Figure 60b). Clearing occurs in approximately a week and a half.

DIAGNOSIS

Although complement fixation tests are available and the virus may be isolated from the feces or throat, the diagnosis is usually made clinically.

DIFFERENTIAL DIAGNOSIS

Most enteroviral exanthems cannot be distinguished from one another on clinical grounds. Herpangina might be confused with a herpetic or candidal infection, but the lesions are usually found in the anterior part of the mouth. There is a high fever. Hand, foot, and mouth disease may have findings similar to those of erythema multiforme. Boston exanthem, caused by echovirus 16, is associated with palmar and plantar pink macules and only mild fever.

TREATMENT

No specific therapy is available.

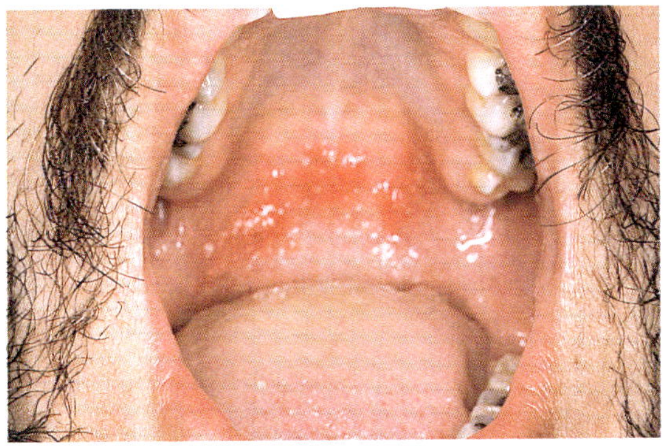

Figure 59
Herpangina shows vesiculopustular ulcerations on the soft palate.

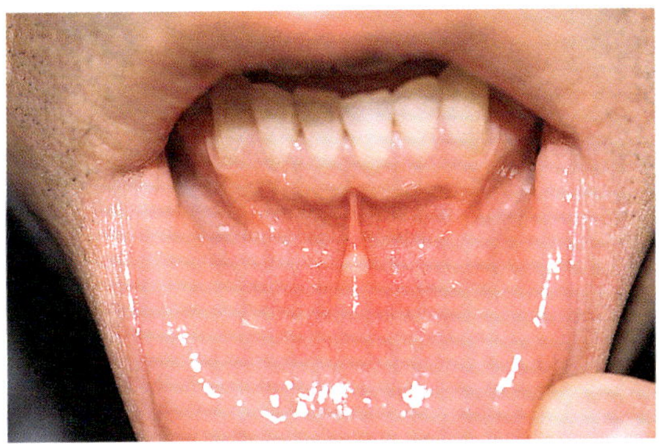

a

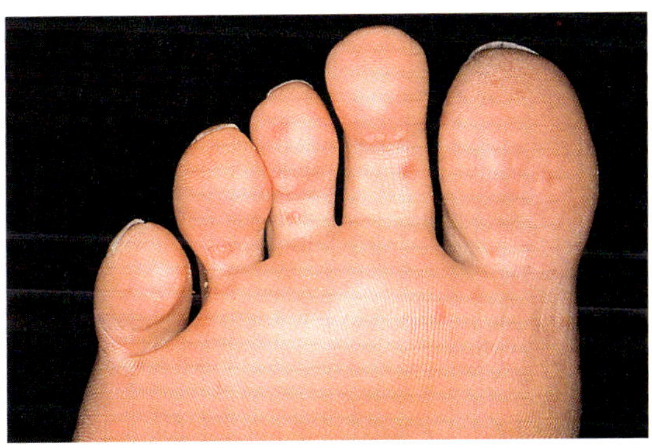

b

Figure 60
Hand, foot, and mouth disease shows (a) small ulcerations on the oral mucosa and (b) angular-shaped vesicles on the toes.

SUGGESTED READINGS

Herbst JS. Exanthems caused by enteroviral infections: coxsackievirus, ECHOvirus, and reovirus: 14–19:1–16. In Demis DJ: Clinical dermatology. Philadelphia, JB Lippincott, 1991.

Russo T, Chang T-W. Eruptions associated with respiratory and enteric viruses. Clin Dermatol 1989;79(1):97–116.

Thomas I, Janniger CK. Hand, foot, and mouth disease. Cutis 1993;52:265–266.

Childhood Exanthems

Six infectious diseases that affect infants and children predominantly have historically been grouped together. Prior to modern laboratory techniques, they were given numbers (Table 8).

ETIOLOGY

The pathogens involved are listed in Table 8.

Table 8 Exanthems of Childhood

Number	Name	Etiologic agent
first disease	measles	measles virus (morbillivirus)
second disease	scarlet fever	ß hemolytic Streptococci, Group A
third disease	rubella	rubella virus (togavirus)
fourth disease	rubella scarlatinosa	unknown
fifth disease	erythema infectiosum	parvovirus B19
sixth disease	exanthema subitum	herpesvirus 6

CLINICAL PRESENTATION

Measles Also known as *rubeola*, is a morbilliform eruption that has an incubation period of about 11 days, during which the catarrhal stage begins. The prodromal period includes conjunctivitis, fever, and the appearance of Koplik's spots, punctate white papules with red halos on the buccal mucosa, opposite the upper molars, lasting up to 2 days. Three days later, the red round to oval lesions begin on the face and spread to involve the whole body, sometimes becoming hemorrhagic. During the next 5 days, there is fever that diminishes as the lesions fade (Figure 61a,b).

Scarlet fever (See Pyogenic Infections.)

Rubella Also called *rötheln* or *German measles*, has an almost silent incubation period of 2 to 3 weeks. The prodromal period of a few days includes mild fever and cervical lymphadenopathy. The maculopapular exanthem starts on the face in the shape of a butterfly and spreads to the entire body. Within 3 days, the eruptions are gone (Figure 62).

Rubella scarlatinosa Occasionally referred to as *Duke's disease*, is said to have small red spots that become confluent and are either rubeoliform or scarlatiniform. There is question of the existence of this disease.

Erythema infectiosum Sometimes called *infectious erythema* or *mégalérythème épidémique*, develops after an incubation period of 6 to 14 days. A figure-of-eight reddening appears on the face, often sparing the mouth. This gives the appearance of having been slapped (Figure 63a). The round to oval erythematous lesions spread to the arms, sometimes presenting as incomplete rings, providing a lacy or reticulated appearance (Figure 63b). The lesions usually clear within hours or by 1 week, leaving no noticeable desquamation. In rare instances, the disease can reappear several times, as seen in one patient whose lesions finally regressed by the ninety-fifth day.

Exanthema subitum Also known as *roseola infantum*, begins 3 to 7 days after the patient is infected. For 3 to 5 days, there is a high fever and malaise. Within hours, the

Figure 61
Measles is characterized by (a) Koplik's spots, discrete yellowish punctate areas on the buccal mucosa, and (b) a morbilliform eruption, blotchy to confluent redness, on the body.

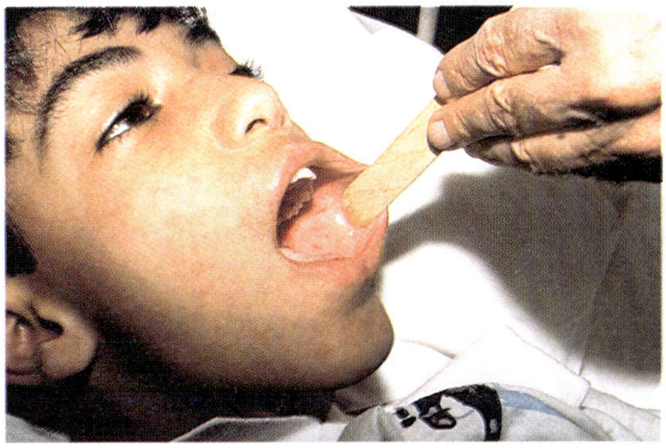

a

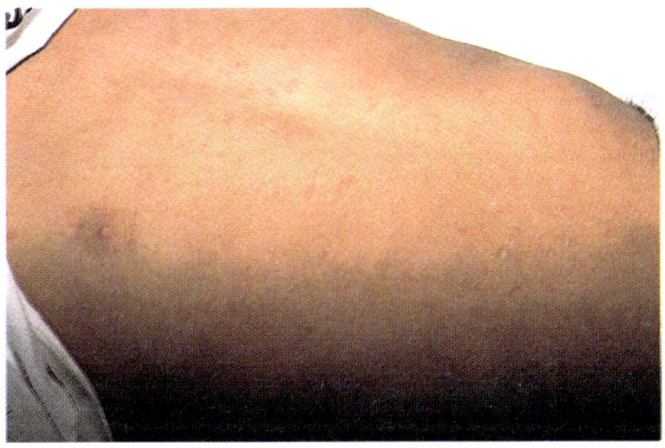

b

Figure 62
Rubella occurred in this young woman who had fever, lymphadenopathy, and a disseminated eruption with tiny erythematous papules.

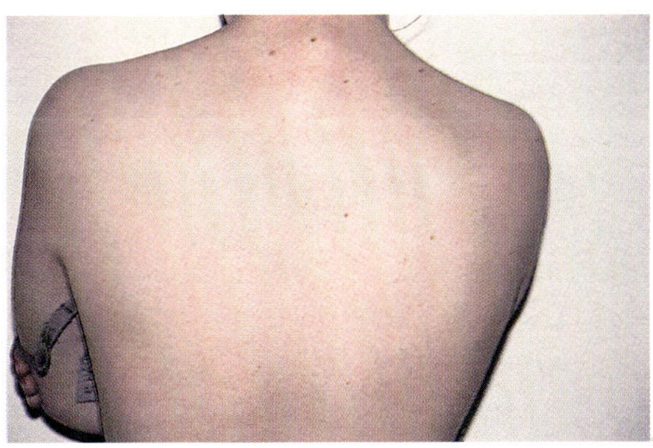

morbilliform eruption appears. It is similar to measles but begins on the trunk. The lesions are 1- to 5-mm pink macules and sometimes papules with a whitish halo. The exanthem spreads, often sparing the face. Within 2 days, it is gone (Figure 64). There may also be edema of the eyelids, red papules on the soft palate and uvula (Nagayama's spots), and even seizures.

DIAGNOSIS

Laboratory tests are generally secondary to clinical observation. Complement fixation titers or ELISA tests can help to confirm some viral infections. Parvovirus B19 may now be detected by IgG and IgM antibodies, identified by Western blot techniques.

DIFFERENTIAL DIAGNOSIS

Many times, the clinical picture is vague enough so that diagnoses such as drug eruptions, vasculitides, atypical mycobacterial infections, and other viral diseases must be considered.

TREATMENT

Except for scarlet fever, for which penicillin or, in penicillin-allergic patients, erythromycin or tetracycline is used, therapy is symptomatic.

SUGGESTED READINGS

Aractingi S, Roujeau JC. Diagnosis of maculopapular rash. Ann Dermatol Venereol 1992;199:307–311.

Asano Y, Yashikawa T, Suga S, et al. Clinical features of infants with primary human herpesvirus 6 infections (exanthem subitum, roseola infantum). Pediatrics 1994;93:104–108.

Bakshi SS, Cooper LZ. Rubella. Clin Dermatol 1989;7(1):8–18.

Bodemer C, de Prost Y. Unilateral laterothoracic exanthem in children: a new disease? J Am Acad Dermatol 1992;27:693–696.

Boyd AS. Laboratory testing in patients with morbilliform viral eruptions. Dermatol Clin 1994;12:69–82.

Chorba T, Anderson LJ. Erythema infectiosum (fifth disease). Clin Dermatol 1989;7(1):65–74.

Hall CB, Long CE, Schnabel KC. Human herpesvirus-6 infection in children: a prospective study of complications and reactivation. N Engl J Med 1994;331:432–438.

Hart CA. Viral redskins. Semin Dermatol 1988;7:48–52.

Höllsberg P, Hafler DA. Pathogenesis of diseases induced by human lymphotropic virus type 1 infection. N Engl J Med 1993;328:1173–1182.

Liebowitz D. Epstein–Barr virus—an old dog with new tricks. N Engl J Med 1995;332:55–56.

Meade RH III. Exanthem subitum (roseola infantum). Clin Dermatol 1989;7(1):92–96.

Neihart RE, Liu C. Measles. Clin Dermatol 1989;7(1):1–7.

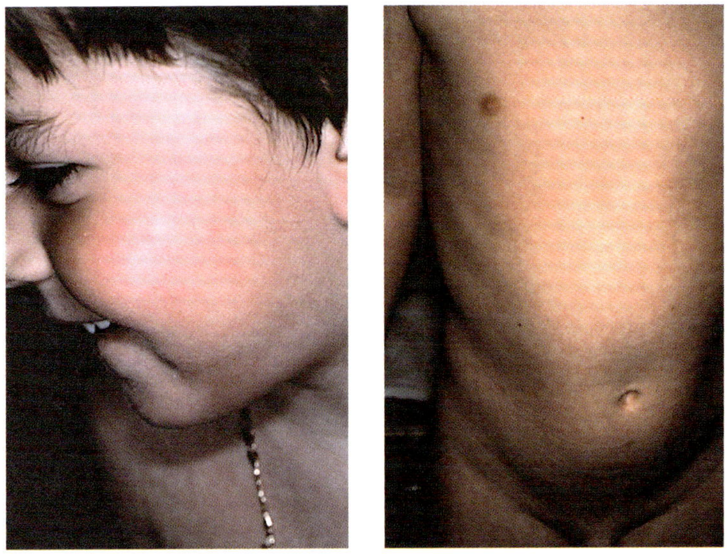

a b

Figure 63
Erythema infectiosum is characterized by (a) the slapped-cheek redness and (b) a figure-of-eight erythematous eruption. (Courtesy of Selim Aractingi, MD, Paris, France.)

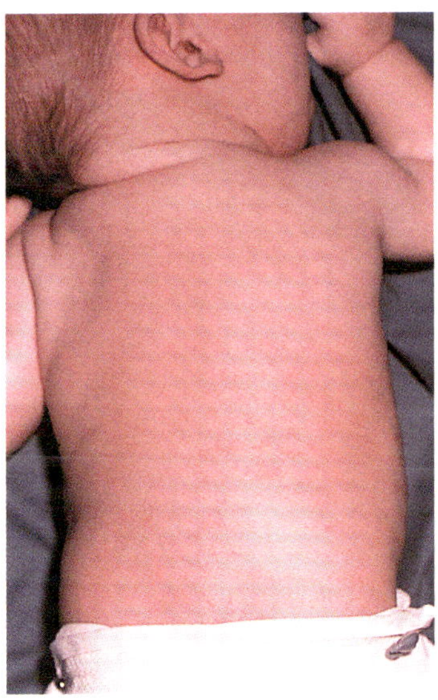

Figure 64
Exanthema subitum was diagnosed in this infant. The diffuse red rash appeared 3 days following the onset of fever.

Acquired Immunodeficiency Syndrome

Acquired immunodeficiency syndrome (AIDS) represents infection with the human immunodeficiency virus (HIV), a retrovirus which permits a host of other infectious agents to cause both common and uncommon conditions. The presentations are generally exaggerated.

ETIOLOGY

HIV enters the body through a break in the skin or mucosa. Within 2 to 16 weeks, it establishes itself in the host, often creating a mononucleosis-like syndrome and eventually leading to AIDS. The primary target of this retrovirus is the CD4+ T-lymphocyte due to its affinity for the CD4 surface marker.

CLINICAL PRESENTATION

Seroconversion may occur anywhere from a few days to 6 months following exposure. The acute retroviral syndrome is characterized by fever, lymphadenopathy, aseptic meningitis, and a maculopapular to confluent eruption (Figure 65a), sometimes resembling pityriasis rosea or infectious mononucleosis (Figure 65b).

Although there are no specific cutaneous manifestations of full-blown AIDS, the presence of several signs are highly suggestive: severe seborrheic dermatitis (Figure 65c), extensive proximal subungual onychomycosis leading to leukonychia (Figure 65d), marked pruritus, eosinophilic folliculitis (Figure 65e), and uncontrolled prurigo nodularis (Figure 65f). The presence of chronic herpes simplex infection, extensive condylomata acuminata, and significant candidosis (Figure 65g) should make the clinician very suspicious. Kaposi's sarcoma is almost pathognomonic of AIDS and may indicate the patient acquired the infection through homosexual activity (Figure 65h). Bacillary angiomatosis and oral hairy leukoplakia similarly are nearly pathognomonic of AIDS or homosexual transmission (Figure 65i).

DIAGNOSIS

The ELISA test is 97% sensitive and the Western blot test is 99% specific in detecting the presence of HIV. Whereas previously the presence of the virus or the disease was classified as persistent, generalized lymphadenopathy (PGL), AIDS-related complex (ARC), and AIDS syndrome (Table 9), the categories are now distinguished by CD4+ and T-lymphocyte counts and symptomatology (Table 10).

Table 9 1986 Classification of HIV Infection

HIV carrier	postive Western blot test, positive ELISA test
PGL	one lymph node with a diameter >1 cm for >3 months, otherwise unexplained
ARC	PGL plus two abnormal laboratory tests and two clinical signs
AIDS	ARC combined with more clinical signs and abnormal laboratory tests

Table 10 1993 Revised Classification of HIV Infection for Adolescents and Adults

CD4+ T-lymphocyte count	A: Asymptomatic, PGL, or acute HIV	B: Symptomatic, not A or C	C: AIDS indicator conditions
≥500/μL	A1	B1	C1
200–499/μL	A2	B2	C2
<200/μL	A3	B3	C3

Category B: bacillary angiomatosis, candidosis (oral, vulvovaginal), cervical dysplasia, fever (38.5°C) or diarrhea, oral hairy leukoplakia, herpes zoster, idiopathic thrombocytopenic purpura, listeriosis, pelvic inflammatory disease, peripheral neuropathy.

Category C: candidosis of bronchi, esophagus, trachea, or lungs; cervical cancer; coccidioidomycosis; cryptococcosis; cytomegalovirus disease; encephalopathy; herpes simplex; histoplasmosis; isopsoriasis; Kaposi's sarcoma; Burkitt's lymphoma; primary lymphoma of the brain; mycobacterial infections (tuberculous or atypical); *Pneumocystis carinii* pneumonia; recurrent pneumonia; progressive multifacial leukoencephalopathy; *Salmonella* septicemia; toxoplasmosis of the brain; wasting syndrome due to HIV.

Adapted from MMWR. Arch Dermatol 1993;129:287–290.

DIFFERENTIAL DIAGNOSIS

The presence of the described dermatologic manifestations is suspicious unless the patient tests negative for HIV.

TREATMENT

In addition to the administration of such drugs as zidovudine (AZT) for the HIV infection, the cutaneous complaints often require imaginative therapy. The fungal infections demand lengthy courses of oral antifungal agents. The bacterial infections need therapy with antimicrobial agents, in addition to the trimethoprim-sulfamethoxasole preparation the patient may already be taking. The dermatoses may call for the use of dapsone or PUVA therapy to control the itching.

SUGGESTED READINGS

Araham A. Aids in the tropics. Dermatol Clin 1994;12:747–752.

Barr CE. Oral diseases in HIV-1 infection. Dysphagia 1992;7:126–137.

Bason MM, Berger TG, Nesbitt LT Jr. Pruritic papular eruption of HIV-disease. Int J Dermatol 1993;32:784–789.

Fisher BF, Warner LC. Cutaneous manifestations of the acquired immunodeficiency syndrome. Int J Dermatol 1987;26:615–630.

MMWR. Arch Dermatol 1993;129:287–290.

Nance KV, Smith ML, Joshi VV. Cutaneous manifestations of acquired immunodeficiency syndrome in children. Int J Dermatol 1991;30:531–539.

Prose NS, Abson KG, Scher RK. Disorders of the nails and hair associated with human immunodeficiency virus infection. Int J Dermatol 1992;31:453–457.

Sadick NS, McNutt NS. Cutaneous hypersensitivity reactions in patients with AIDS. Int J Dermatol 1993;32:621–627.

Spach DH. Bacillary angiomatosis. Int J Dermatol 1992;31:19–24.

Warner LC, Fisher BF. Cutaneous manifestations of the acquired immunodeficiency syndrome. Int J Dermatol 1986;25:337–350.

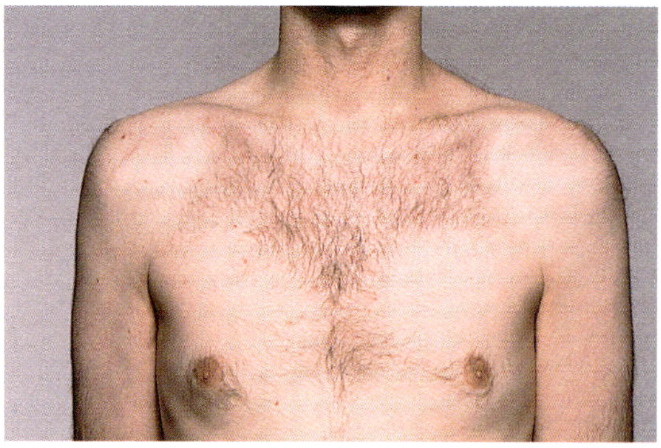

a

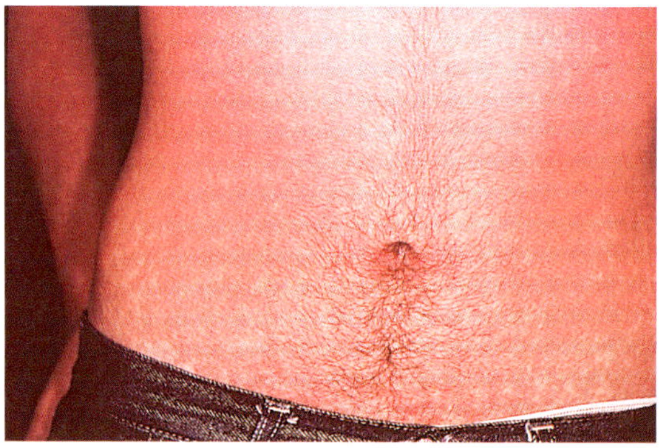

b

Figure 65
AIDS may first be diagnosed at the time of seroconversion (a) when there is a blotchy erythematous eruption. This patient's eruption on his chest and neck took 2 months to clear. (Courtesy of David A Hawkins, FRCP (UK), London, England.) (b) The clinical picture may be similar to infectious mononucleosis, which could be distinguished by a monospot test. (c) Severe seborrheic dermatitis and (d) proximal subungual onychomycosis might suggest the diagnosis. (Courtesy of Antar Padilha-Gonçalves, MD, Rio de Janeiro, Brazil.) (e) Eosinophilic folliculitis, which is characterized by papules, nodules, and excoriations and (f) prurigo nodularis, with scaling and excoriated nodules (Courtesy of Antar Padilha-Gonçalves, MD, Rio de Janeiro, Brazil.) should also make the clinician suspicious. (g) Thrush in a debilitated patient and the appearance of (h) Kaposi's sarcoma with its typical purplish macules and plaques or (i) hairy leukoplakia with white papular lesions on the lateral surface of the tongue all point toward a diagnosis of immunodeficiency.

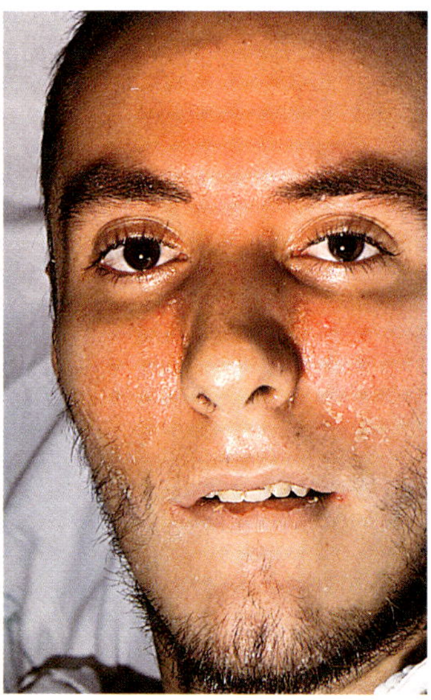

c

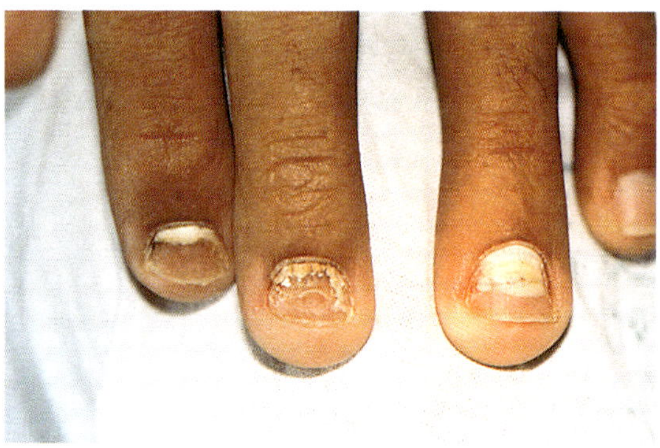

d

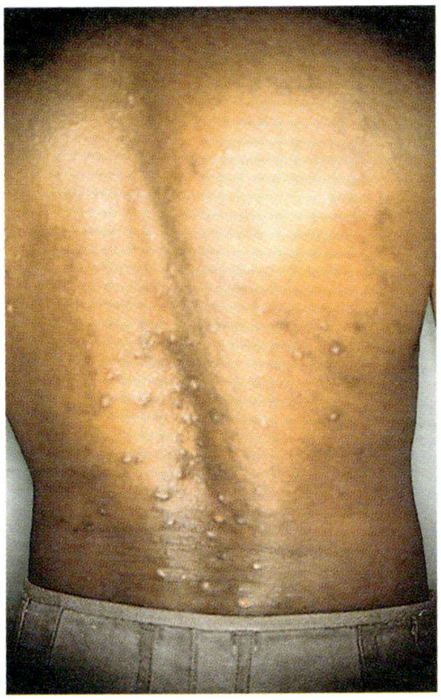

e

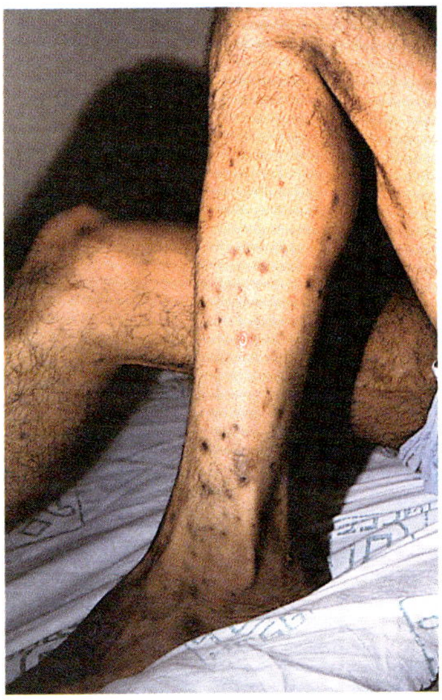

f

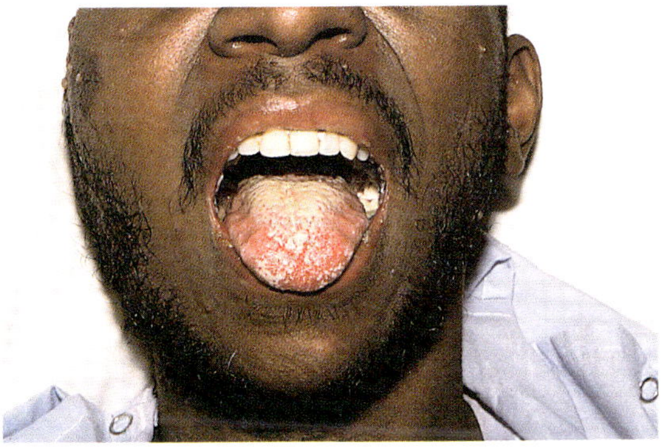

g

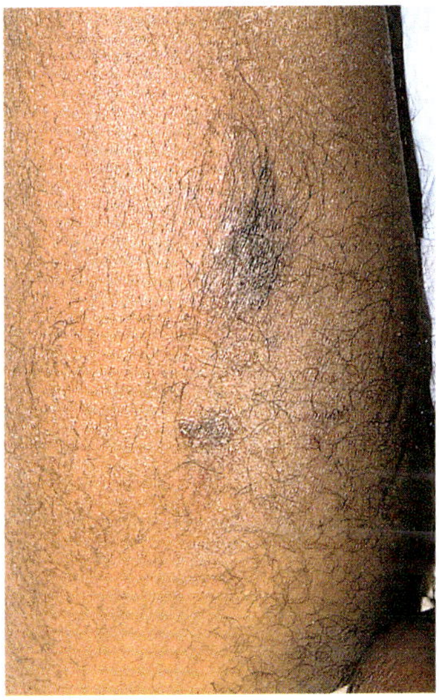

h

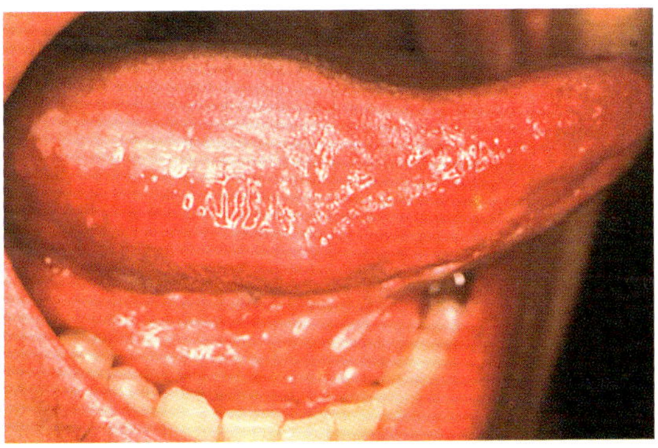

i

SUPERFICIAL FUNGAL INFECTIONS

Dermatophytes

Dermatophytes live in the stratum corneum or other structures rich in keratin, such as nails and hair. Rarely do they penetrate deeper into the skin. They can be categorized as zoophilic (found in animals), including *Microsporum canis*; geophilic (found in soil), including *Microsporum gypseum* or *Trichophyton mentagrophytes*; and anthrophilic (found in humans), including *Epidermophyton floccosum*, *Trichophyton rubrum*, and *Trichophyton tonsurans*.

Tinea Capitis

Tinea capitis, or ringworm of the scalp, reaches epidemic proportions among children at various times, whereas tinea barbae occurs infrequently today.

ETIOLOGY

Infection of scalp hair is commonly caused by *Trichophyton tonsurans*, *Microsporum audouinii*, *M. canis*, and *T. verrucosum*. *T. schoenleinii* causes an unusual infection known as favus. Children who are most often afflicted contract the fungi by person-to-person contact, from animals, or from fomites.

CLINICAL PRESENTATION

Gray-patch tinea capitis Well-defined circular areas of alopecia with scaling and broken-off hairs, close to the surface of the scalp. It is most often caused by *M. audouinii* and *M. canis*, which remain on the hair shaft (ectothrix) (Figure 66a).

Black dot tinea capitis Few to numerous, ill-defined small scaly patches of incomplete hair loss. The affected hairs break off within the follicles, so that they give the appearance of black dots. It is most often caused by *T. tonsurans* and *T. violaceum*, which invade the hair shaft (endothrix) (Figure 66b).

Kerion formation Boggy inflammatory process due to bacterial infection accompanying the fungal infection. The hairs fall out or can be pulled easily. The site is red, edematous, painful, and prone to scarring (Figure 66c).

Favus Severely scarring process caused most often by *T. schoenleinii* and less often by *T. quinkeum, T. mentagrophytes, T. violaceum* and *M. gypseum*. There are small yellowish crusts with elevated borders and depressed centers, called *scutula*. The red exudative areas coalesce to form large plaques and emit a rat-like odor. Cervical lymphadenopathy is common. Occasionally, lesions may be found on the skin (Figure 66d,e).

Tinea barbae Well-defined circular areas of erythema and scaling with hairs being broken off close to the skin surface. Follicular papules, pustules, and even kerion formation complete the picture. *T. mentagrophytes* and *T. verrucosum* are most often implicated (Figure 66f).

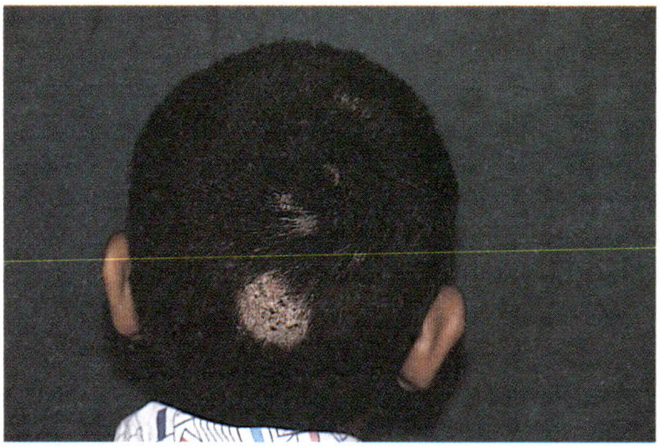

a

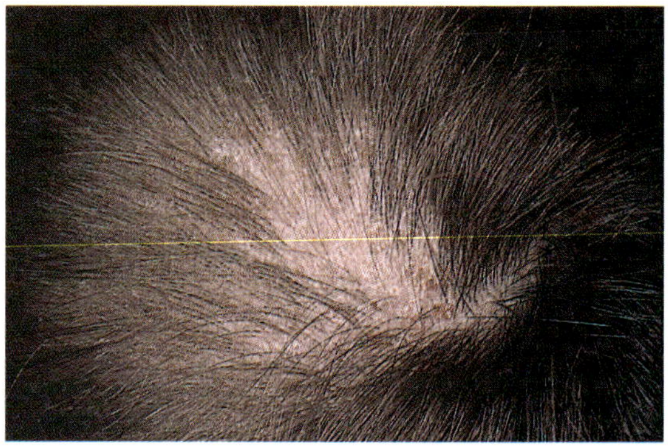

b

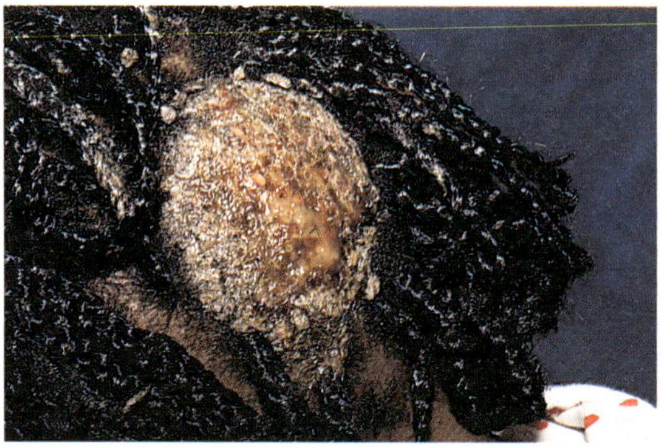

c

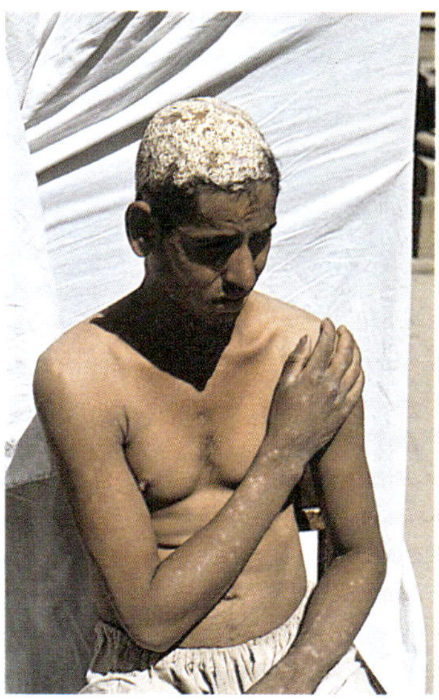

d

Figure 66
Tinea capitis may appear as (a) the gray-patch type due to *M. canis*, in which there is scaling and broken hairs or as (b) the black dot type due to *T. tonsurans*, in which the broken hairs appear as dark specks on the scalp. (c) A kerion, being a boggy inflammatory mass, represents secondary bacterial infection or hypersensitivity. Favus, characterized by yellowish crusting with elevated borders (scutula), occurs usually on the scalp (d), but occasionally, a scutula can be seen on the arm (e). (Courtesy of Mohsen Sollimon, MD, Cairo, Egypt.) (f) Tinea barbae can be extremely painful, as shown in this patient with crusting, oozing, and marked inflammation. (Courtesy of Guy Chabeau, MD, Lyon, France.)

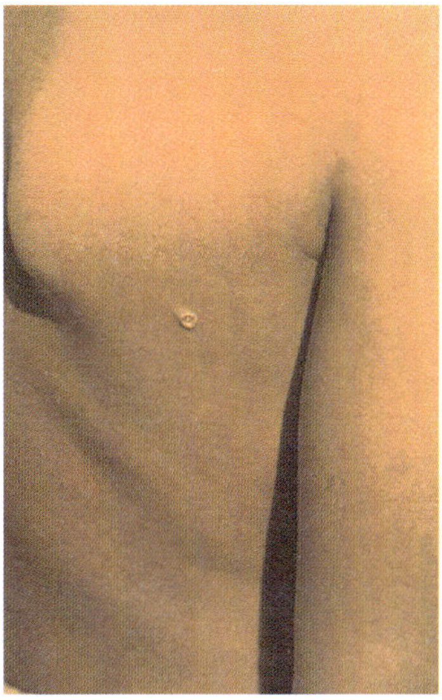

e

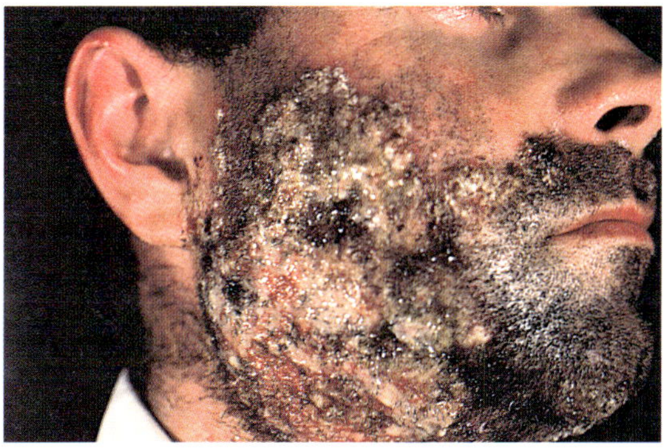

f

DIAGNOSIS

Wood's light examination will reveal greenish fluorescence of hairs infected by ectothritic fungi, *M. audouinii*, and *M. canis*, whereas *T. schoenleinii* fluoresces a grayish green. The more common pathogens today *T. tonsurans* and *T. violaceum*, being endothritic, do not fluoresce. Culture of the hairs and scalp scale on appropriate media will reveal the organism.

DIFFERENTIAL DIAGNOSIS

Traditionally, alopecia areata and seborrheic dermatitis have been confused with tinea capitis. Tinea barbae may be similar to pyoderma. Fungal and bacterial cultures will help in making the diagnosis.

TREATMENT

Fungal infections of the hair follicles require the use of systemic agents. Creams, solutions, and shampoos sometimes are useful adjuvants, but they do not replace the necessary oral agents (Table 11).

Table 11 Agents Useful in Treating Fungal Infections

Agent	Administration		
Historical agents			
dyes			
Castellani's paint	topical		
gentian violet	topical		
keratolytic			
Whitfield's ointment	topical		
miscellaneous			
potassium iodide		oral	
undecylenic acid	topical		
Older agents			
8-hydroxyquinoline			
iodochlorhydroxyquin	topical		
penicillium			
griseofulvin		oral	
halogenated phenol			
haloprogin	topical		
thiocarbamate			
tolnaftate	topical		
Newer agents			
polyene antibiotics			
nystatin	topical	oral*	
amphotericin B	topical		parenteral
pyrimidine			
flucytosine		oral	
imidazoles			
bifonazole	topical		
clotrimazole	topical		
econazole	topical		
ketoconazole	topical	oral	
miconazole	topical		parenteral
oxiconazole	topical		
sulconazole	topical		
tioconazole	topical		
triazoles			
fluconazole		oral	
itraconazole		oral	
terconazole	topical		
morpholine			
amorolfine	topical		
hydroxypyridone			
ciclopiroxolamine	topical		
allyamines			
naftifine	topical		
terbinafine	topical	oral	

*No systemic absorption.

SUGGESTED READINGS

Al-Fouzan AS, Nanda A, Kubec K. Dermatophytosis of children in Kuwait: a prospective survey. Int J Dermatol 1993;32:798–801.

Cauwenbergh G. Antifungal therapy. In: Parish LC, Millikan E, Amer M, et al, eds. Global Dermatology. New York: Springer-Verlag, 1994:317–330.

Crissey JT, Lang H, Parish LC. Manual of Medical Mycology. Cambridge: Blackwell Science, 1995:1–263.

Gupta AK, Sauder DN, Shear NH. Antifungal agents: an overview. J Am Acad Dermatol 1994;30:677–698, 911–933.

Hays AG, Buntin DM, Wible LO. Black dot tinea capitis in man. Int J Dermatol 1993;32:740–742.

Herbert AA. Tinea capitis: current concepts. Arch Dermatol 1988;124:1554–1557.

Lee JY, Hsu ML. Tinea capitis in adults in southern Taiwan. Int J Dermatol 1991;30:572–575.

Moore MK, Suite M. Tinea capitis in Trinidad. J Trop Med Hyg 1993;96:346–348.

Pursley TV, Raimer SS. Tinea capitis in the elderly. Int J Dermatol 1980;19:220.

Stiller MJ, Sanqueza OP, Shupack JL. Systemic drugs in the treatment of dermatophytoses. Int J Dermatol 1993;32:16–21.

Verenkar MP, Pinto MJ, Rodrigues SJ, et al. Tinea capitis due to *Trichophyton schoenleinii*. Indian J Pathol Microbiol 1991;34:299–301.

Vidimos AT, Camisa C, Tomecki KJ. Tinea capitis in three adults. Int J Dermatol 1991;30:206–208.

TINEA CORPORIS

Tinea corporis represents a fungal infection of the glabrous skin.

ETIOLOGY

T. rubrum is the most commonly isolated organism at present. Other fungi often recovered from the skin are *T. mentagrophytes*, *T. tonsurans*, and *M. canis*, particularly when there are pets in the household. Other molds, such as *Scytalidium* species, are being identified as pathogens.

CLINICAL PRESENTATION

Tinea corporis Can have several presentations usually associated with mild pruritus. There may be well-defined, ovoid to circular, red, elevated, scaling rings with central clearing, particularly with *M. canis*, or erythematous, concentric scaling rings or red scaling patches with polycyclic borders and no tendency for central clearing when *T. rubrum* is the pathogen. Scaling plaques with pustules suggest *T. mentagrophytes* infection (Figure 67a).

Tinea faciei Indicates that the fungal infection is limited to the face (Figure 67b). A special variety is tinea incognito, in which the repeated applications of topical steroids to the face or other parts of the body allows the fungus to proliferate. Many clinical manifestations are reduced by the anti-inflammatory properties of the steroid (Figure 67c).

Tinea cruris Known as *jock itch*, may be defined as tinea corporis limited to the crural region and genitalia (Figure 67d).

Tinea imbricata Also called *tokelau*, it is characterized by scaling, concentric, annular to polycyclic rings covering the trunk and extremities. The causative agent is *T. concentricum*, the only Trichophyton not to invade hair. It is seen in southeast Asia, the South Pacific islands, Central and South America, and South Africa (Figure 67e).

Majocchi's granuloma Represents invasion of the hair follicles, usually on the legs. There are follicular papules and pustules on ill-defined scaling patches. It occurs following minor trauma from friction, maceration, or shaving (Figure 67f).

DIAGNOSIS

KOH scrapings and fungal cultures will confirm the clinical suspicion.

DIFFERENTIAL DIAGNOSIS

A variety of dermatitides, ranging from pityriasis rosea and nummular dermatitis to psoriasis, granuloma annulare, and erythema annulare, may mimic tinea corporis. Tinea cruris appears similar to candidosis but no satellite lesions or maceration is present. Erythrasma is differentiated by its coral-red fluorescence produced by the Wood's light. Tinea imbricata has often been confused with a variety of ichthyoses.

TREATMENT

Both oral and topical treatment can be recommended.

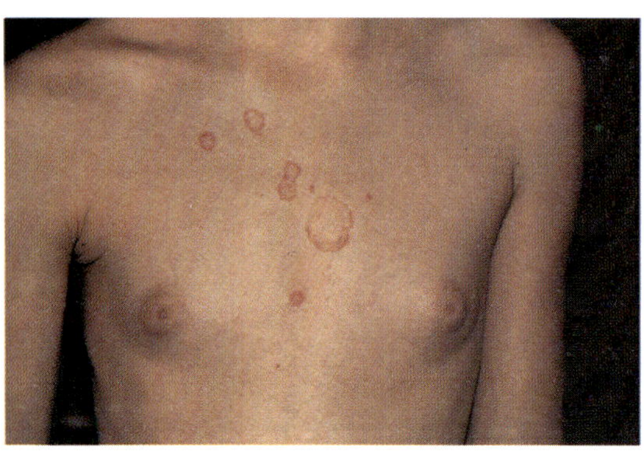

a

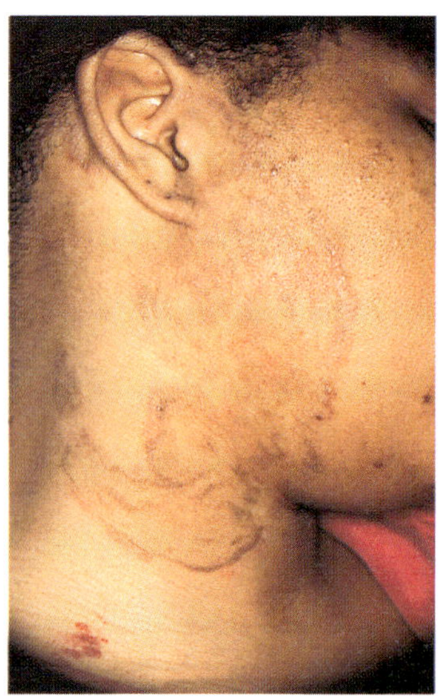

b

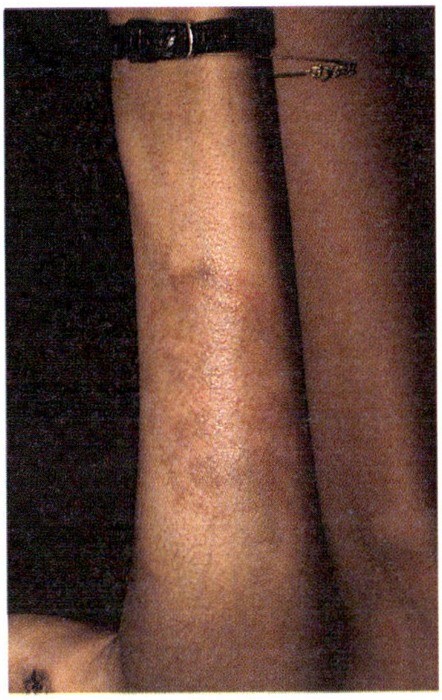

c

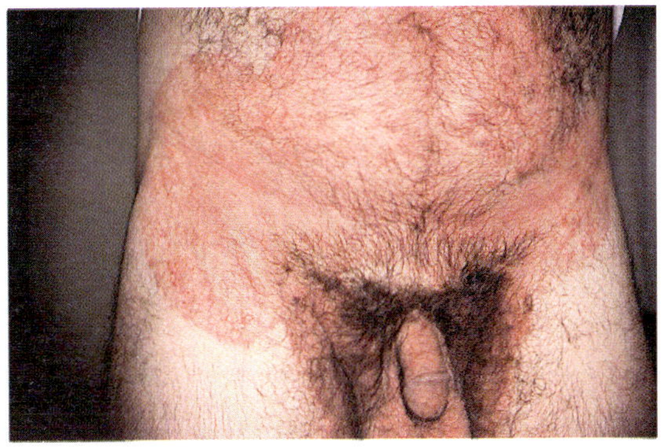

d

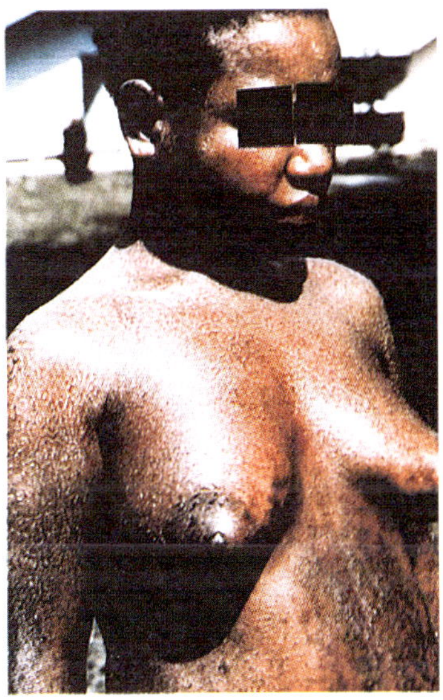

e

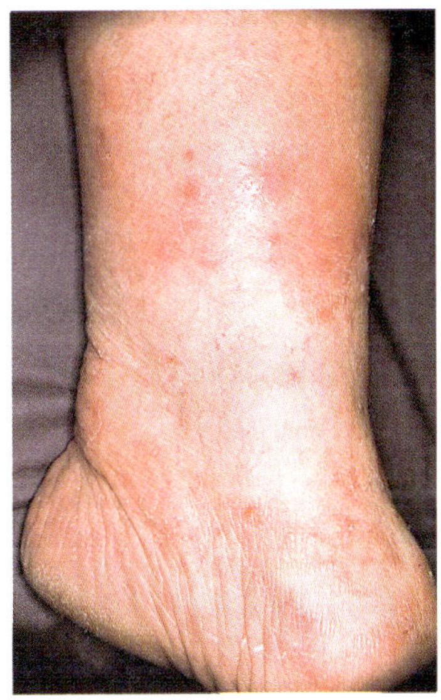

f

Figure 67
(a) Tinea corporis often has annular red lesions with central clearing. (b) This patient with tinea faciei has a more intense inflammatory reaction. (c) Topical steroids can mask a fungal infection initially, but rapid growth of the dermatophyte leads to the characteristic redness and scaling known as *tinea incognito*. (d) This patient had such extensive inflammation with redness and scaling that diagnoses of tinea corporis and tinea cruris could be made. (e) Tinea imbricata is composed of concentric rings extending out over the skin. (f) Majocchi's granuloma occurred as a result of leg shaving.

SUGGESTED READINGS

Cox NH, Irving B. Cutaneous "ringworm" lesions of *Scopulariopsis brevicaulis*. Br J Dermatol 1993;129:726–728.

Degreef H. The treatment of superficial skin infections caused by dermatophytes. Curr Top Med Mycol 1992;4:189–206.

Elewski BE, Hazen PG. The superficial mycoses and the dermatophytes. J Am Acad Dermatol 1989;21:655–673.

Foil CS. Fungal diseases. Clin Dermatol 1994;12:529–547.

Ghorpade A, Ramanan C. Tinea capitis and corporis due to *Trichophyton violaceum* in a six-day-old infant. Int J Dermatol 1994;33:219–220.

Macura AB. Primer of dermatology: dermatophyte infections. Int J Dermatol 1993;32: 313–323.

Moore MK. The infection of human skin and nail by *Scytalidium species*. Curr Top Med Mycol 1992;4:1–4.

TINEA PEDIS

Tinea pedis, also called *athlete's foot*, was almost unknown in the nineteenth century.

ETIOLOGY

A number of dermatophytes, including *T. rubrum, T. mentagrophytes, Epidermophyton floccosum*, and even *T. tonsurans* in children who have tinea capitis, have been implicated. *Candida albicans*, a pseudoyeast, and such saprophytes as *Scytalidium dimidiatum* and *S. hyalinum*, can cause infection on the feet. Moisture and occlusion are necessary ingredients for this type of infection.

CLINICAL PRESENTATION

Dermatophytosis simplex The mildest form of tinea pedis, characterized by scaling of the interdigital web with occasional fissuring. The fourth interspace usually is involved. The condition is usally asymptomatic but may be associated with mild intermittent pruritus (Figure 68a).

Dermatophytosis complex Maceration, denudation, and erythema of the toe webs and opposing sides in the severe form. It may be mild (Figure 68b) or severe (Figure 68c). The toes of the fourth interspace and occasionally the third are involved. There is some thickening of the interdigital skin, giving a whitish appearance in the mild form. There is itching and the presence of a foul odor.

Gram-negative athelete's foot Occurs in a small number of patients where there is the addition of inflammation and edema. The erythema extends to the dorsal surface of the toes and feet. There is denudation of the interspaces, sides of the toes, and plantar surface. A serous or purulent discharge usually is present. The condition frequently involves the second, third, and fourth interspaces (Figure 68d).

Acute vesicobullous infection A recurrent, highly inflammatory condition in which vesicles arise on the arch, heel, and interdigital area. The lesions may be isolated or become confluent to form bullae, filled with clear, sticky fluid. When they break, there is a painful base. Secondary bacterial infection or immunologic reaction to the fungi may lead to cellulitis, lymphangitis, or lymphadenitis. Between acute inflammatory episodes, the involved areas show low-grade scaling. An id reaction may appear on the hands (Figure 68e).

Id reaction In severe forms of tinea pedis, there is enough inflammatory reaction that dermatitis occurs elsewhere, usually on the hands. No fungi have ever been recovered at the site of this allergic response (Figure 68f).

Chronic mocassin-type infection Characterized by diffuse scaling on the soles. This may be patchy or involve the entire weight- bearing surface. Hyperkeratosis may be limited to the heels and sides of the feet. The infection usually is asymptomatic, with painful fissures generally developing in the elderly. The nails may be involved. Often, this leads to the one-hand, two-feet syndrome (Figure 68g).

DIAGNOSIS

KOH scrapings and fungal cultures will confirm the clinical suspicion.

DIFFERENTIAL DIAGNOSIS

Contact dermatitis, atopic dermatitis, and psoriasis sometimes are confused with tinea pedis. The topography and morphology can be so similar that differentiation may require several observations.

TREATMENT

Topical agents are often useful. However, in the more severe forms of *T. rubrum* infection, particularly the mocassin foot, oral antifungal agents are needed. Ciprofloxacin, 500 mg PO bid, is required for gram-negative athelete's foot syndrome.

SUGGESTED READINGS

Dahl MV. Suppression of immunity and inflammation by products produced by dermatophytes. J Am Acad Dermatol 1993;28:S19–23.

Macura AB. Dermatophyte infections. Int J Dermatol 1993;32:313–323.

Miller MA, Hodgson Y. Sensitivity and specificity of potassium hydroxide smears of skin scrapings for the diagnosis of tinea pedis. Arch Dermatol 1993;129:510–511,1342–1343.

Nishimoto K. The presence of dermatophytes in the environment and on healthy looking skin: their significance as a cause of disease in Japan. Curr Top Med Mycol 1993;5:201–214.

Stiller MJ, Shupack JL, Rosenthal SA. Treatment of dermatophytosis II: newer topical antifungal drugs. Int J Dermatol 1993;32:638–641.

Witkowski JA, Lemont H. Color atlas of cutaneous disorders of the lower extremities. New York: Igaku-Shoin, 1993:1–127.

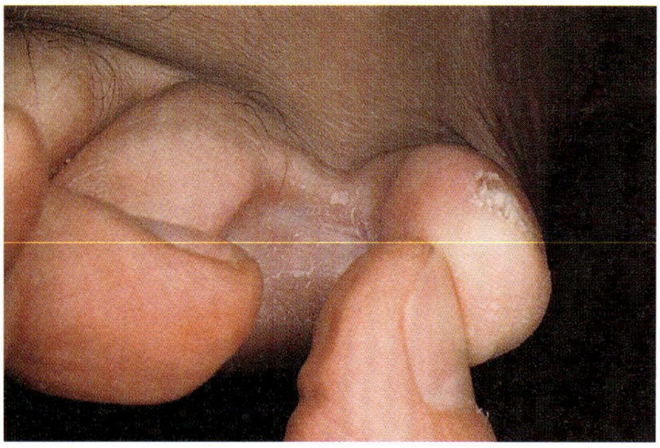

a

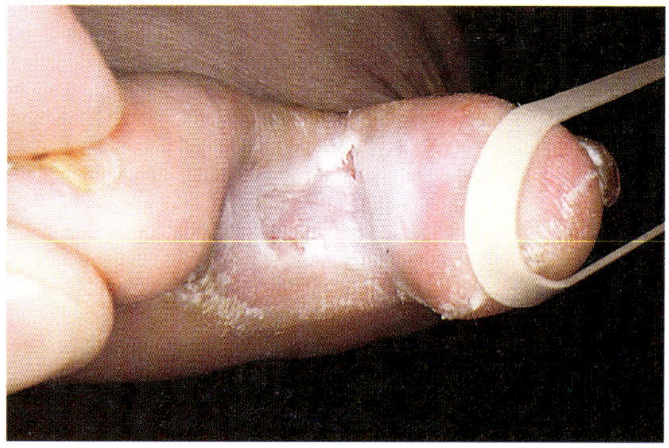

b

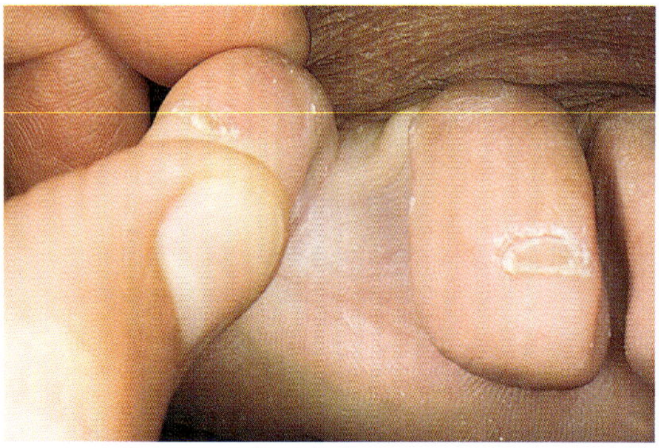

c

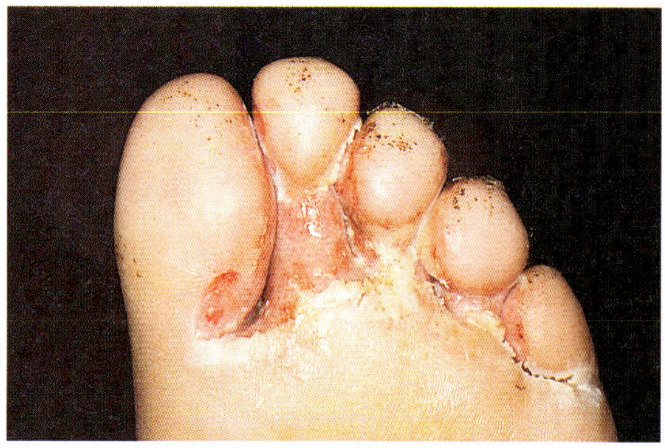

d

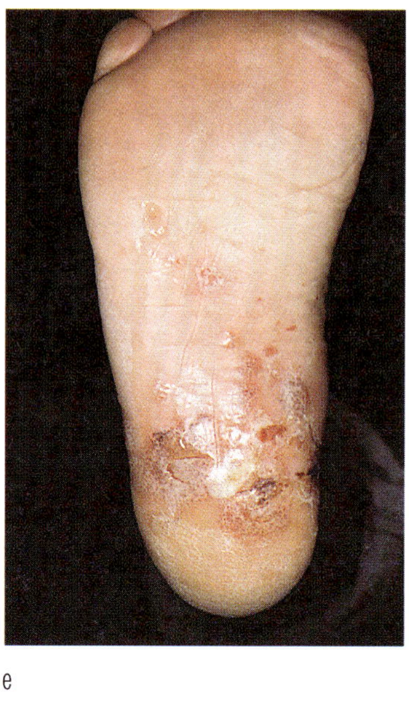

e

Figure 68
Tinea pedis may present as (a) dermatophytosis simplex or as (b,c) dermatophytosis complex. (d) Gram-negative athlete's foot is more erosive and painful. (e) The acute vesiculobullous infection may create a red, crusted, and sore dermatitis. (f) With severe infections, an id reaction, characterized by papules and vesicles, may appear on the hands. (g) The mocassin type of fungal infection, so-called because it looks like a shoe covering, is most often due to *T. rubrum* infection.

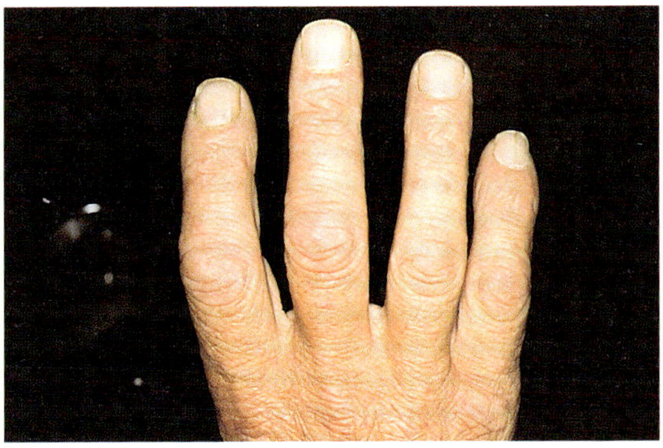

f

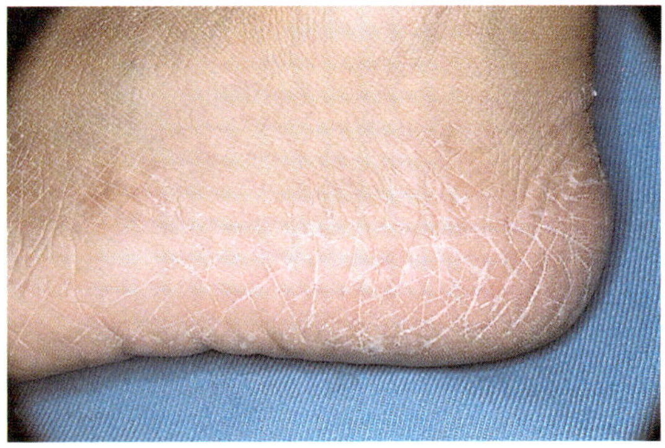

g

Onychomycosis

Onychomycosis is an increasing problem that causes much embarrassment to patients.

ETIOLOGY

At one time, *T. rubrum* and, less commonly, *E. floccosum* and *T. mentagrophytes*, were believed to be the only pathogens. Currently, several other organisms are accepted as causing dystrophy of the nails: *Scytaldium dimidiatum*, *S. hyalinum*, *Scopulariopsis brevicaulis*, molds, and *C. albicans*.

CLINICAL PRESENTATION

Fungal infection of the nails may have four presentations.

Distal subungual type Characterized by whitish, yellow, or tan discoloration of the edge of the nail with subungual keratinous debris (Figure 69a).

White superficial type Identified by the presence of well-defined white spots on the nail plate. These may enlarge and coalesce to create a rough surface (Figure 69b).

Proximal subungual type Characterized by whitening under the proximal part of the nail plate. This occurs most often on the toenails. When it appears on the fingernails, the clinician should have a high suspicion of acquired immune deficiency syndrome (AIDS) (Figure 69c).

Candida onychomycosis Associated with chronic paronychia of the involved digit. The nail dystrophy begins centrally or laterally and spreads distally over the nail plate. Fingernails usually are involved. Pain in the nail bed is a frequent complaint, and there is onycholysis, ridging, and discoloration (Figure 69d).

DIAGNOSIS

KOH scrapings and fungal cultures will confirm the clinical suspicion.

DIFFERENTIAL DIAGNOSIS

Fungal infections often spare several nails, and this would differentiate onychomycosis from a systemic disease such as psoriasis. Traumatic nail disease would more likely show ridges and afflict a few nails. Discoloration occurs with bacterial nail infections (Figure 69e,f).

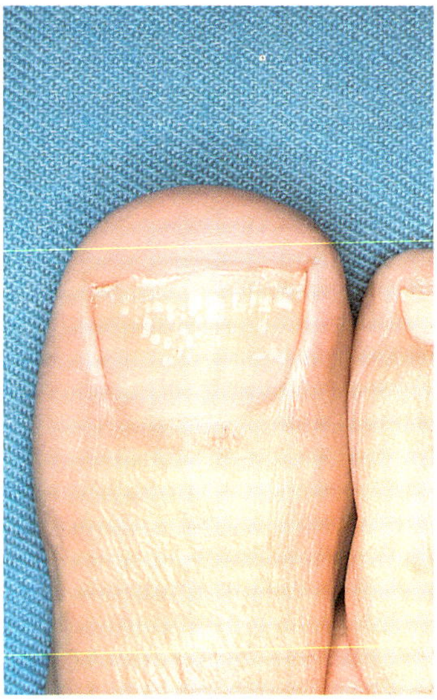

a

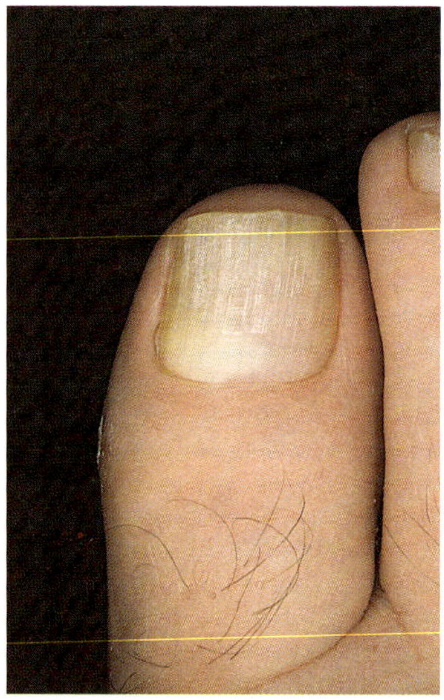

b

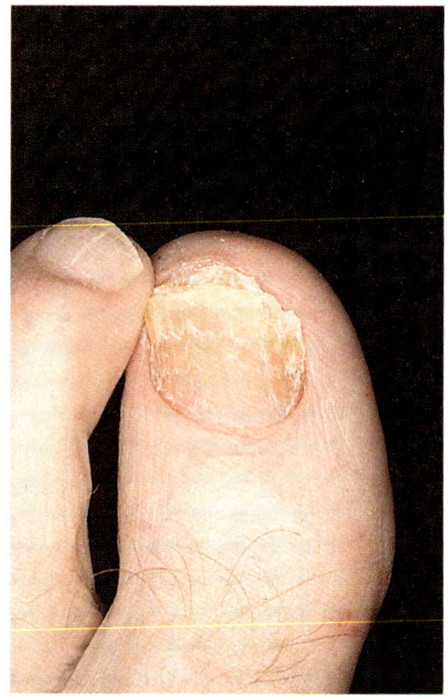

c

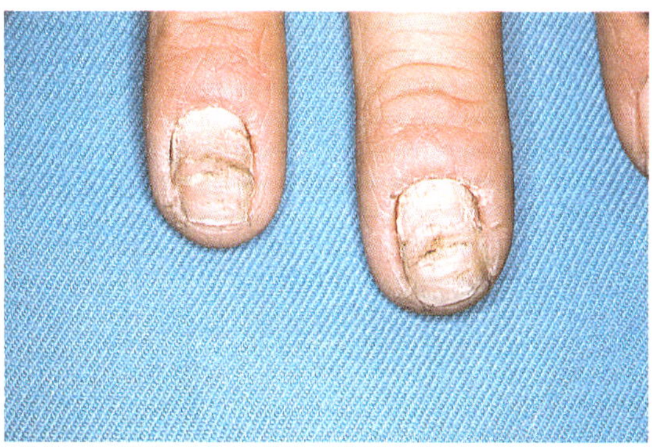

d

Figure 69
Onychomycosis may present as (a) a brittle, yellowish nail or (b) with more debris and proximal whitening. (c) With stippling, the nail may be described as *leukonychia trichophytica*. (d) This patient also had a monilial paronychia that led to the destruction of the nail. (e) Infection with *Pseudomonas aeruginosa* creates greenish discoloration, whereas (f) infection with Proteus species gives a brownish black color.

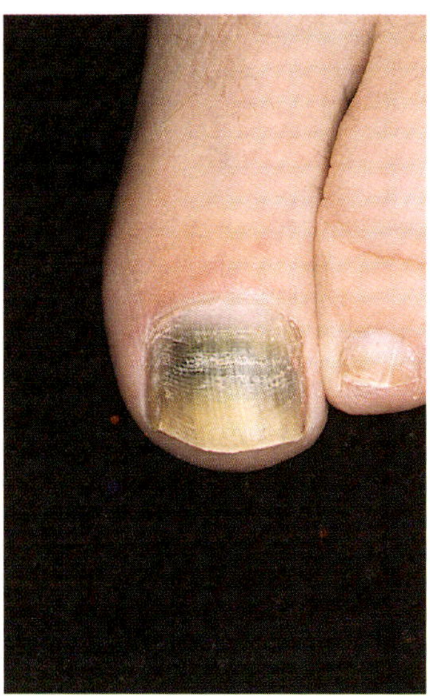

e

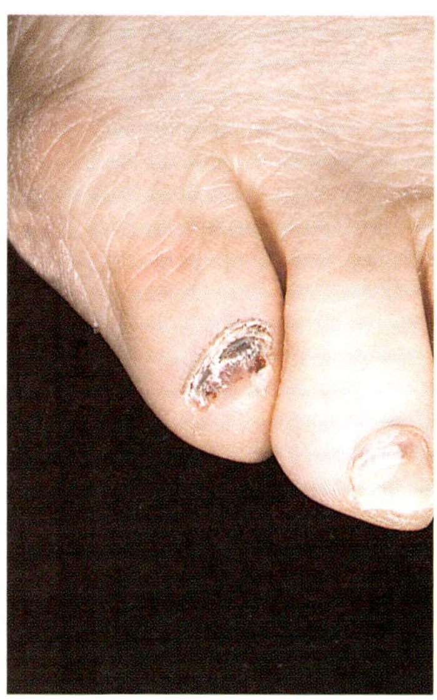

f

TREATMENT

Although several topical formulations, even as nail lacquers, are under investigation, current management involves the use of oral antifungal therapy. Fluconazole, itraconazole, and terbinafine are so well absorbed and have such affinity for keratin that they may be given for short periods of time, whereas griseofulvin and ketoconazole require many months of therapy.

SUGGESTED READINGS

André J, Achten G. Onychomycosis. Int J Dermatol 1987;26:481–490.

Baran R. Nail disease. Semin Dermatol 1991;10:1–87.

Hanke E. Fungal infections of the nail. Semin Dermatol 1991;10:41–53.

Piérard GE, Arrese JE, Pierre S, et al. Diagnostic microscopique des onychomyoses. Ann Dermatol Venereol 1994;121:25–29.

Prose NS, Abson KG, Scher RK. Disorders of the nails and hair associated with human immunodeficiency virus infection. Int J Dermatol 1992;31:453–457.

Roberts D. Fungal nail infections. Practitioner 1993;237:22–26.

Roseeuw D, DeDoncker P. New approaches to the treatment of onychomycosis. J Am Acad Dermatol 1993;29:S45–50.

Schafer-Korting M. Pharmacokinetic optimisation of oral antifungal therapy. Clin Pharmacokinet 1993;25:329–341.

YEAST-LIKE ORGANISMS

Yeast-like organisms cause a variety of skin manifestations, generally very superficial, but sometimes more extensive.

CANDIDOSIS

Candidosis is the disease created by members of the genus Candida. While immune deficiency and metabolic diseases such as diabetes mellitus permit more yeast infection, many other patients also suffer from infection caused by Candida species.

ETIOLOGY

Candida albicans is the most common cause of candidosis. It is often found in the gut and in the vagina, as it prefers a warm, moist environment. The intertriginous and mucocutaneous areas are preferred sites. Less commonly, other types of Candida create disease: *C. guilliermondii, C. krusei, C. pseudotropicalis, C. tropicalis,* and *C. stellatoidea*.

CLINICAL PRESENTATION

Candidal infections generally create a reddened area, sharp borders, and satellite lesions. Several distinctive forms are known.

Oral candidosis (thrush) A disease of infants, older patients, and the immunocompromised, characterized by white papules and patches on the buccal mucosa and tongue. When the lesions are scraped, the base is found to be raw and eroded. In newborns, the mothers are often found to have vaginal candidosis (Figure 70a,b).

Vulvovaginitis and balanitis Grayish white to reddish patches on the genitalia, often accompanied by marked itching (Figure 70c). In women, there may be a creamy white discharge (Figure 70d).

Pseudoblastomyces interdigitale Erythema and scaling that is found in the finger webs (Figure 70e).

DIAGNOSIS

The clinical picture may be confirmed by a KOH scraping and positive fungal culture.

DIFFERENTIAL DIAGNOSIS

Fungal studies will differentiate oral candidosis from oral hairy leukoplakia, lichen planus, and geographic tongue. Candidal infection elsewhere on the body may be confused with a dermatophyte infection or contact dermatitis.

TREATMENT

Nystatin topicals or inserts have been used effectively for decades. The newer antifungal agents can be recommended topically and as inserts. For more extensive infections, the administration of the new oral agents can be prescribed.

SUGGESTED READINGS

Almeida Santos L, Beceiro J, Hernandez R, et al. Congenital cutaneous candidosis: report of four cases and review of the literature. Eur J Pediatr 1991;150:336–338.

Coleman DC, Bennett DE, Sullivan DJ, et al. Oral Candida in HIV infection and AIDS: new perspectives /new approaches. Crit Rev Microbiol 1993;19:61–82.

Fotos PG, Ray TL. Oral and perioral candidosis. Semin Dermatol 1994;13:118–124.

Thomas I. Superficial and deep candidosis. Int J Dermatol 1993;32:778–783.

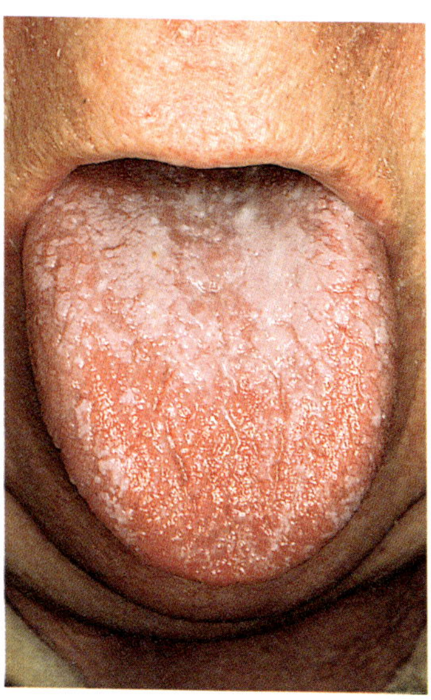

a

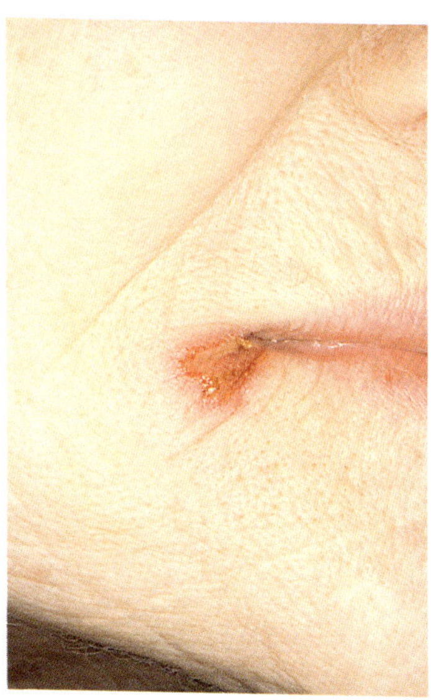

b

Figure 70
Candidosis may present as (a) whitish coating on the tongue (thrush) or as (b) red scaling at the commissure (perleche). (c) Candidal balanitis may appear as diffuse redness on the penile shaft, whereas (d) candidal vulvovaginitis may also extend to thighs and demonstrate the characteristic satellite lesions of *C. albicans* infection. (e) Pseudoblastomyces interdigitale is an expensive name for candidal infection of the finger webs.

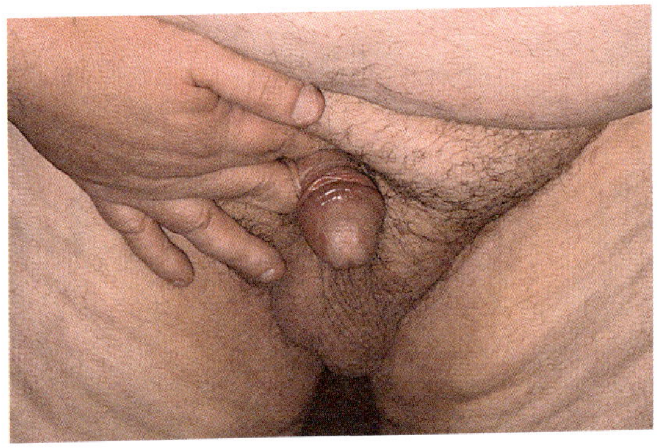

c

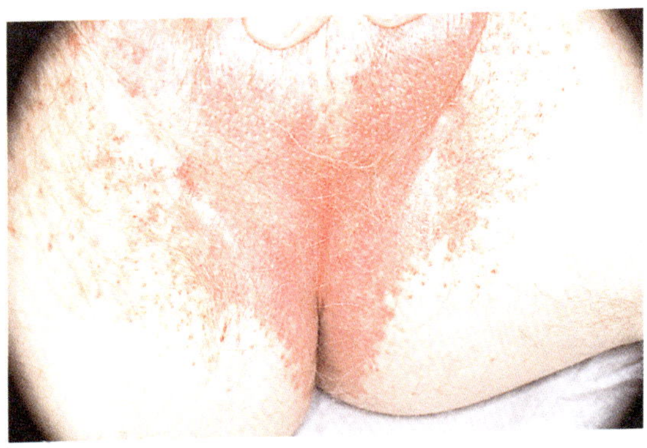

d

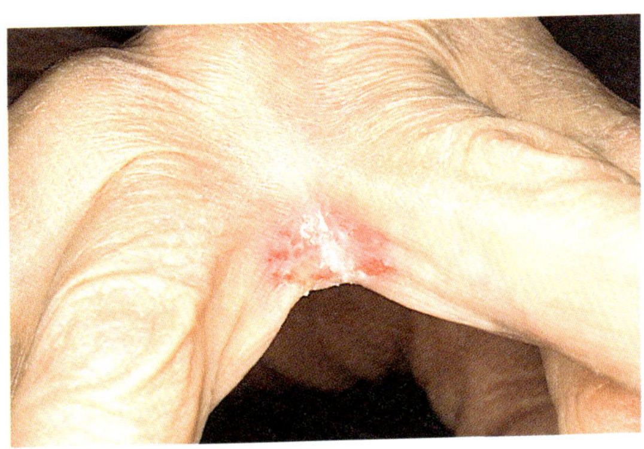

e

Chronic Mucocutaneous Candidosis

Chronic mucocutaneous candidosis (CMC), also called *monilial granuloma, candida granuloma*, and *granulomatous candidosis*, is a recurrent infection of the skin, mucous membrane, and nails. It occurs in association with polyendocrinopathy, interstitial keratitis, and thymomas.

ETIOLOGY

Patients with CMC have T cells that are unable to respond to *Candida* antigens and fail to produce lymphokines such as gamma interferon.

CLINICAL PRESENTATION

The initial lesion is usually thrush with angular cheilitis. The cutaneous involvement begins with brown dry scaling or erythematous skin on the face, scalp, ears, neck, and shoulders. In severe cases, hyperkeratotic crusted lesions are found on the face and scalp, where osteolytic lesions are known to develop. The lesions have the appearance of horns (Figure 71). The fingernails are usually involved. Although the hair is not involved, scarring alopecia often occurs.

DIAGNOSIS

The clinical picture may be confirmed by a KOH scraping and positive fungal culture. Histopathologic examination may show the granulomatous formation. Intradermal skin tests with candidal antigen are usually negative at 48 hours.

DIFFERENTIAL DIAGNOSIS

Acrodermatitis enteropathica, seborrheic dermatitis, psoriasis, and dermatophytosis may have similar manifestations.

TREATMENT

In addition to long-term therapy with itraconazole, 200 mg daily, or fluconazole, 400 mg on day one and then 200 mg daily, adjunctive measures are usually needed. These include the use of transfer factor, thymosin, cimetidine, or levamisole.

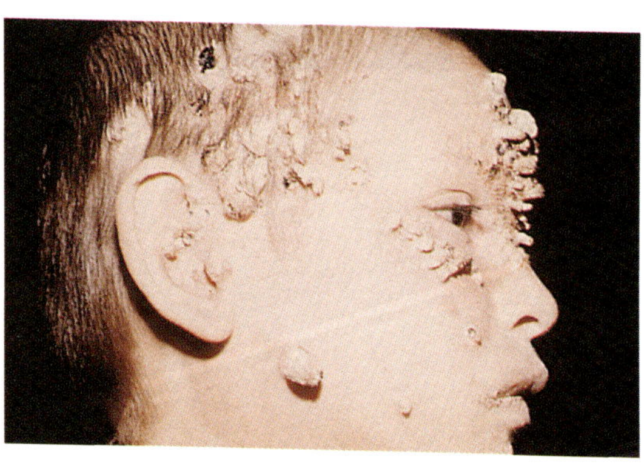

Figure 71
The lesions of chronic mucocutaneous candidosis are often hyperkeratotic and crusted. (Courtesy of Sebastião AP Sampãio, MD, São Paulo, Brazil.)

SUGGESTED READINGS

Mateev G, Kantardjiev T, Vassileva S, et al. Chronic mucocutaneous candidosis with osteolysis of the frontal bone. Int J Dermatol 1993;32:888–889.

Noh LM, Hussein SH, Sukumaran KD, et al. Chronic mucocutaneous candidosis with deficient CD2 (E receptor) but normal CD3 mononuclear cells. J Clin Lab Immunol 1991;35:89–93.

Ro BI. Chronic mucocutaneous candidosis. Int J Dermatol 1988;27:457–462.

Pityrosporum Ovale Infections

Pityrosporum ovale infections include tinea versicolor and pityrosporum folliculitis. The organism may play a causal role in confluent and reticulated papillomatosis and seborrheic dermatitis.

ETIOLOGY

The genus Pityrosporum (*Malassezia*) includes the lipophilic yeasts *Pityrosporum orbiculare* and *P. ovale*. They are part of the normal flora of the hair follicle. Apparently, increased numbers result in clinical manifestations and a transformation of the yeast form to the hyphal form. Enzymes metabolize the skin lipids to produce dicarboxylic acids that inhibit tyrosinase and are toxic to melanocytes. This results in hypopigmentation of the affected sites. Clinical manifestations seem to appear more commonly when there is a depression in the cellular immunity.

CLINICAL PRESENTATION

Tinea versicolor (pityriasis versicolor) Hypopigmented to hyperpigmented patches of skin with scaling, usually appearing on the trunk but sometimes elsewhere on the body (Figure 72a,b,c).

Pityrosporum folliculitis Pruritic, follicular red papules and pustules, usually on the trunk (Figure 72d).

Confluent and reticulated papillomatosis (Gougerot-Carteaud syndrome) Grayish brown papules that coalesce to form a rough or verrucous surface, which may have a reticulated or confluent configuration. The lesions are often found on the trunk, beginning on the presternum and spreading elsewhere (Figure 72e).

Seborrheic dermatitis Redness and scaling, often with sharp borders, found on the scalp, glabella, paranasal area, submentum, sternum, axillae, umbilicus, groin, and the intergluteal cleft.

DIAGNOSIS

Clinical suspicion can be confirmed by a KOH scraping, which will show hyphae and budding cells. Exposed areas of skin may fluoresce a greenish color.

DIFFERENTIAL DIAGNOSIS

Because the diseases are mild and scaling, they may be confused with a drug eruption, neurodermatitis, and psoriasis.

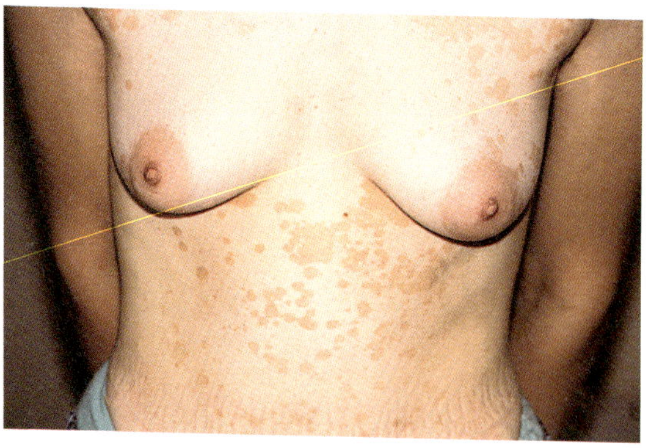

a

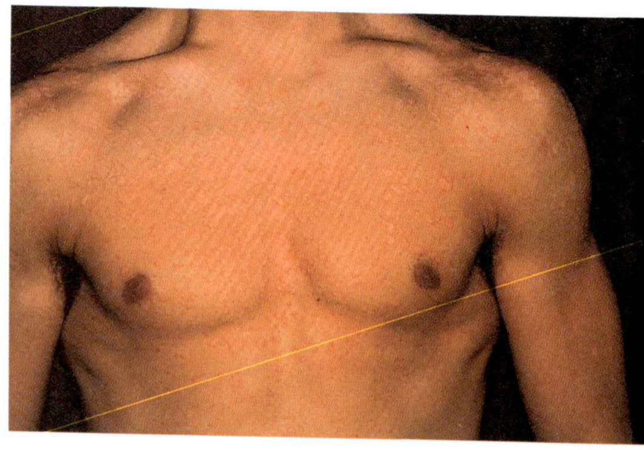

b

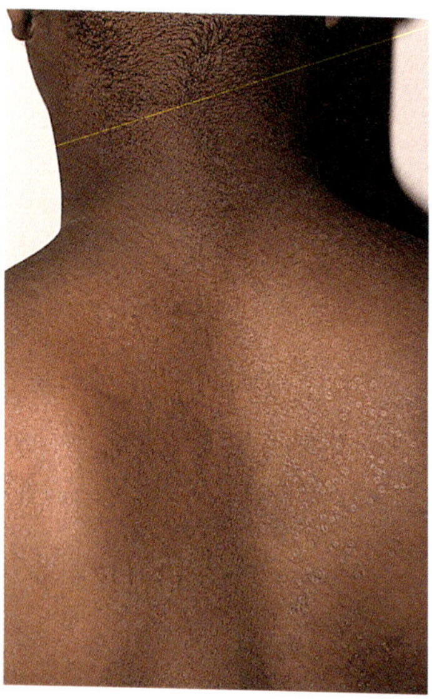

c

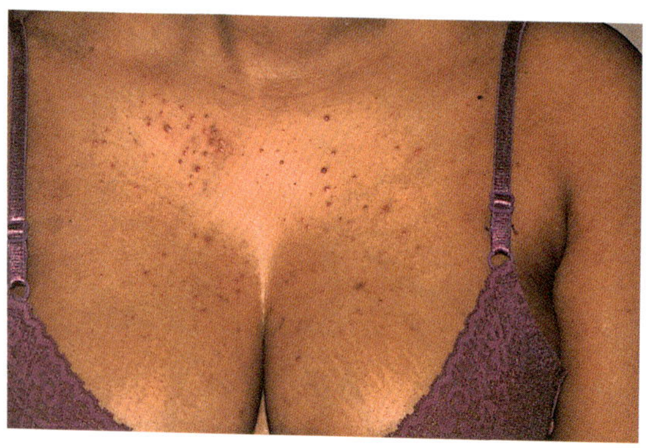

d

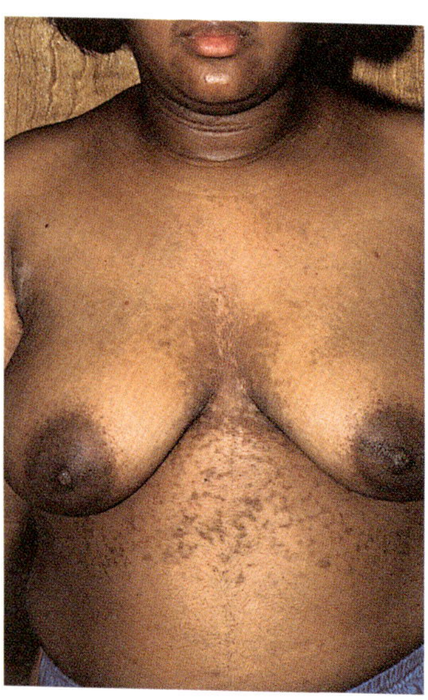

e

Figure 72
(a,b,c) *Pityrosporum ovale* infections are commonly seen as tinea versicolor, so-called because of the many colors it creates depending upon the color of the patient's skin and the exposure to sunlight. (d) *Pityrosporum* folliculitis is nonspecific until it is distinquished through microscopic examination of the contents of a pustule. (e) Confluent and reticulated papillomatosis is characterized by lines of hyperpigmentation and some scaling.

TREATMENT

With the advent of the new triazoles, a short course of oral therapy—itraconazole, 100 mg bid for 7 to 10 days—will eliminate tinea versicolor. However, frequent relapses are found. Topical antifungal agents applied for 3 to 4 weeks can also be used. Whitfield's ointment is acceptable for the treatment or small areas.

Pityrosporum folliculitis may be treated with topical or oral medication, whereas confluent and reticulated papillomatosis lends itself more to the use of oral agents.

SUGGESTED READINGS

Ashbee HR, Ingham E, Holland KT, et al. The carriage of *Malassezia furfur* serovars A, B and C in patients with pityriasis versicolor, seborrhoeic dermatitis and controls. Br J Dermatol 1993;129:533–540.

Faergemann J. Epidemiology and ecology of pityriasis versicolor. Curr Top Med Mycol 1989;3:153–167.

Faergemann J. *Pityrosporum ovale* and skin diseases. Keio J Med 1993;42:91–94.

Patel SD, Noble WC. Analyses of skin surface lipid in patients with microbially associated skin disease. Clin Exp Dermatol 1993;18:405–409.

Payle B, Serrano L, Bieley HC, et al. Albert's solution versus potassium hydroxide solution in the diagnosis of tinea versicolor. Int J Dermatol 1994;33:182–183.

Shrum JP, Millikan LE, Bataineh O. Superficial fungal infections in the tropics. Dermatol Clin 1994;112:687–693.

Sykes NL. Earwax and tinea versicolor. Int J Dermatol 1994;33:543–544.

SUBCUTANEOUS FUNGAL INFECTIONS

Dimorphous fungi commonly are found in decaying vegetation or the soil and usually produce disease after trauma. They also have the propensity for creating infections, predominantly in the subcutaneous tissue.

Sporotrichosis

Sporotrichosis is a chronic granulomatous and ulcerative infection of both humans and animals. Its distribution is worldwide.

ETIOLOGY

The growth of *Sporothrix schenckii* is favored by high humidity and warm temperatures. The fungus gains entry into the host as a result of trauma. Gardeners are particularly prone to this infection as a result of pricks from rose or barberry thorns, sphagnum moss, or straw.

CLINICAL PRESENTATION

Approximately 3 weeks after the trauma, at the site of inoculation, a small red, firm, nontender subcutaneous nodule appears. The lesion gradually becomes violaceous and breaks down to form an ulcer with a ragged, necrotic base. Sporotrichosis then progresses in one of three ways. Most commonly, there is proximal advancement with nodules developing along a lymphatic chain, usually along an arm. They enlarge and ulcerate (sporotrichoid pattern) (Figure 73a). Less commonly, when the lesion is on the face or abdomen, it may enlarge and ulcerate in the localized area (Figure 73b). Rarely, there is hematogenous dissemination to skin, bones, joints, lungs, genitourinary tract, eyes, and meninges.

DIAGNOSIS

Growth on fungal medium will identify the organism, whereas histologic examination of the lesion often shows nonspecific changes.

DIFFERENTIAL DIAGNOSIS

A sporotrichoid pattern can be seen in leishmaniasis and atypical mycobacterial infections. Tularemia and cutaneous tuberculosis sometimes can have similar presentations. Appropriate cultures and histologic study should reveal the correct diagnosis.

TREATMENT

With the introduction of the second-generation oral antifungal agents, the treatment has been simplified. Itraconazole, 200 mg daily, for nearly a month, can be prescribed. Previously, saturated solution of potassium iodide was used. The initial dose of 5 drops tid is given, with an increase to 40 drops tid. This is continued for a month after clearing. Isolated lesions are sometimes excised.

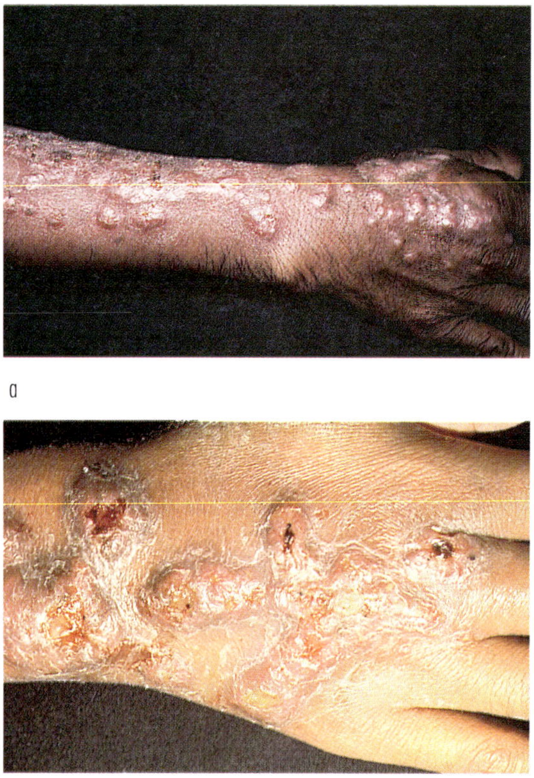

a

b

Figure 73
(a) Sporotrichosis often appears as a chain of nodules, as in this 63-year-old man who contracted the infection 3 months earlier. (b) Sometimes the lesions coalesce, as they did in this 27-year-old woman who had sporotrichosis for 6 months. (Courtesy of Roberto Arenas, MD, Mexico City, Mexico.)

SUGGESTED READINGS

Gumaa SA. Sporotrichosis. In: Mahgoub E-S, ed. Tropical Mycoses. Beerse, Belgium: Janssen Research Council, 1991:149–159.

Itoh M, Okamoto S, Karlya M. Survey of 200 cases of sporotrichosis. Dermatologica 1986;172:209–213.

Mercurio MG, Elewski BE. Therapy of sporotrichosis. Semin Dermatol 1993;12:285–289.

Purvis RS, Diven DG, Drechsel RD, et al. Sporotrichosis presenting as arthritis and subcutaneous nodules. J Am Acad Dermatol 1993;28:879–884.

Werner AH, Werner BE. Sporotrichosis in man and animal. Int J Dermatol 1994;33:692–700.

Chromomycosis

Chromomycosis is a polymorphic fungal infection with a propensity for the legs of men, particularly farm workers in the tropics.

ETIOLOGY

Five fungi account for most infections described as chromomycosis: *Fonsecaea pedrosoi, F. compactum, Phialophora verrucosa, Cladosporium carrioni,* and *Rhinocladiella aquaspersa*. The infection usually starts with a puncture wound that allows the fungus to enter the skin.

CLINICAL PRESENTATION

The infection begins as a pink papule that expands to form nodules and tumors with smooth, hyperkeratotic or verrucous surfaces. The lesions are often covered with foul-smelling crusts and epidermal debris. Peripheral extension often results in central healing with atrophic scars, leading to annular, arciform, or serpiginous lesions. The lateral surface of the foot is commonly affected, and the area often is very pruritic (Figure 74).

Secondary infection and satellite lesions occur after scratching and autoinoculation. Sometimes, the superficial lymphatics are also responsible for satellite lesions. When lymphatic obstruction occurs, there may be elephantiasis. Rarely, there may be hematogenous spread, which permits abscess formation at distant sites, even the brain.

DIAGNOSIS

KOH examination of skin scrapings containing the black dots may show the pathognomonic "copper pennies." Cultures will reveal the pathogen, whereas histologic studies will show pseudoepitheliomatous hyperplasia, granulomatous infiltrate, and the fungi within the giant cells.

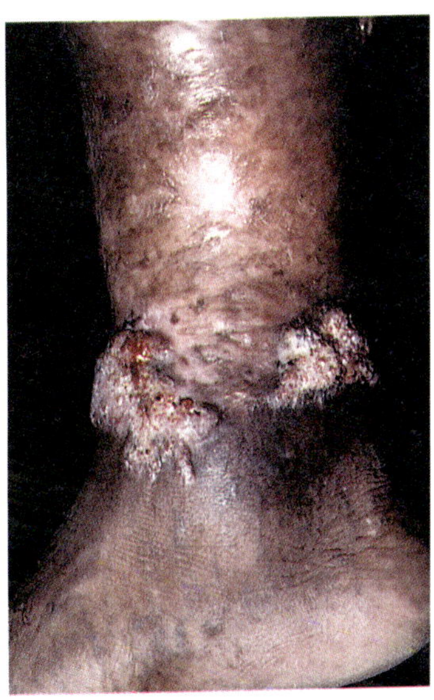

Figure 74
Chromomycosis is characterized by hypertrophic, verrucous, crusted lesions. (Courtesy of Antar Padilha-Gonçalves, MD, Rio de Janeiro, Brazil.)

DIFFERENTIAL DIAGNOSIS

Deep fungal infection, such as blastomycosis, leprosy, leishmaniasis, cutaneous tuberculosis, and bromoderma, may resemble chromoblastomycosis.

TREATMENT

For isolated lesions, surgical intervention by cold steel, liquid nitrogen, or laser can be used. More extensive involvement requires the use of 5-fluorocytosine, 200 mg/kg/day PO, or amphotericin B, 0.5 mg/kg/day IV. Ketoconazole has also been used in dosages of 200 to 400 mg daily.

SUGGESTED READINGS

Beardmore GL. Chromomycosis and phaehypomycosis. In: Mahgoub E-S, ed. Tropical Mycoses. Beerse, Belgium: Janssen Research Council, 1991:75–91.

Gross ML, Millikan LE. Deep fungal infections in the tropics. Dermatol Clin 1994;12:695–700.

Hiruma M, Ohbishi Y, Ohat H, et al. Chromomycosis of the breast. Int J Dermatol 1992;31:184–185.

MYCETOMA

Mycetoma, also known as *Madura foot*, is a chronic granulomatous disease that usually affects the skin and subcutaneous tissue but sometimes involves the fascia, muscle, and bone.

ETIOLOGY

The disease may be caused by such aerobic bacteria (actinomycetoma) as *Nocardia brasiliensis*, *N. asteroides*, *Actinomadura madurae*, *A. pelletieri*, and *Streptomyces somaliensis*, or by such true fungi (eumycetoma) as *Madurella grisea*, *Pseudoallescheria boydii*, *Leptospheria senegalensis*, and species of Acremonium. The organisms penetrate the foot. Typical patients are men working the fields in the tropics who may injure a foot on a thorn or wood splinter.

CLINICAL PRESENTATION

The affected site becomes a hard, painless tumefaction with nodules, abscesses, and fistulas developing. There is drainage of seropurulent to serosanguineous exudate containing granules or grains characteristic of the infectious agents (Figure 75).

DIAGNOSIS

Material is examined microscopically for granules after it has been softened by KOH and pressure is applied to the coverslip for flattening. Material for culturing and histologic examination should be taken deeply from the area surrounding a sinus tract. Histologically, there may be microabscesses and a granulomatous pattern. X-rays show areas of bone lysis and production.

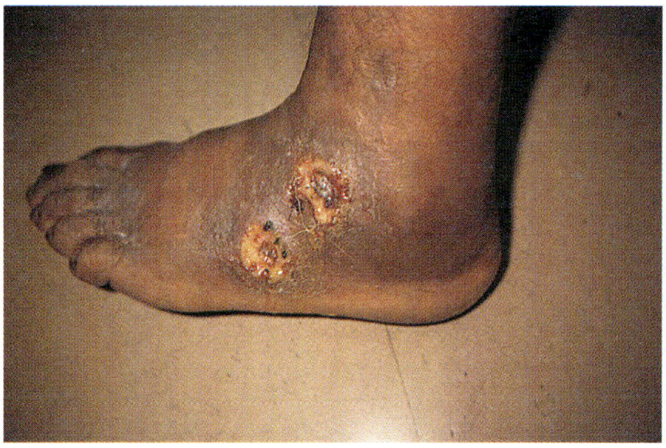

Figure 75
Mycetoma is described as having ulcerations and draining sinuses.

DIFFERENTIAL DIAGNOSIS

Botryomycosis, tuberculosis, osteomyelitis, and even malignant tumors may resemble a mycetoma.

TREATMENT

Therapy depends on finding the causative organism. Frequently, trimethoprim-sulfamethoxazole is used for 6 months following clinical cure. Itraconazole, 200 to 400 mg/day for a similar period, can be used for mycetoma of fungal origin.

SUGGESTED READINGS

Dixon DM, Polak-Wyss A. The medically important dermatiaceous fungi and their identification. Mycoses 1991;34:1–18.

Hay RJ, Mahgoub ES, Leon G, et al. Mycetoma. J Med Vet Mycol 1992;30(suppl 1):41–49.

Magaña M. Mycetoma. Int J Dermatol 1984;23:221–236.

Mahgoub E-S. Mycetoma. In: Mahgoub E-S, ed. Tropical mycoses. Beerse, Belgium: Janssen Research Council, 1991:57–74.

Welsh O. Mycetoma: current concepts in treatment. Int J Dermatol 1991;30:387–398.

Welsh O. Mycetoma. Semin Dermatol 1993;12:290–295.

Lobomycosis

Lobomycosis, also called *keloid blastomycosis* and *Jorge Lobo's disease*, is a chronic disease resulting in keloid formation.

ETIOLOGY

Paracoccidioides loboi is the suspected pathogen, although it has not been cultured. The infection occurs in men working in the Brazilian Amazon, although dolphins and the six-banded armadillos have also become infected. The skin is usually traumatized by animal or insect bites.

CLINICAL PRESENTATION

The disease is found on exposed areas, particularly the ears. It appears as a freely movable nodule that enlarges peripherally to form a large plaque. The surface becomes lobulated or verucoid but rarely ulcerates. Through autoinoculation, satellite lesions appear. The lesions are occasionally mildly pruritic (Figure 76).

DIAGNOSIS

Histologic study will show characteristic dermal granulomas with giant cells that contain yeast cells having multiple branching points and buds in chains. KOH scrapings can suggest the diagnosis stated above.

DIFFERENTIAL DIAGNOSIS

Diseases that cause keloid formation, such as tuberculosis verrucosa cutis, leishmaniasis, chromomycosis, and lepromatous leprosy, can have similar presentations.

TREATMENT

Because there is no effective medical therapy, surgical excision or cryosurgery is recommended.

SUGGESTED READINGS

Borelli D. Lobomycosis. In: Mahgoub E-S, ed. Tropical mycoses. Beerse, Belgium: Janssen Research Council, 1991:161–173.

Gross ML, Millikan LE. Deep fungal infections in the tropics. Dermatol Clin 1994;12:695–700.

Rodrigues-Toro G. Lobomycosis. Int J Dermatol 1993;32:324–332.

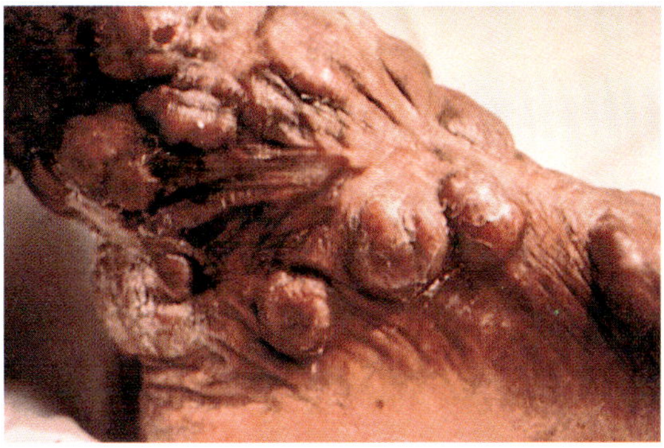

Figure 76
Lobomycosis represents massive keloid formation. (Courtesy of F. Soland, MD, San José, Costa Rica.)

Rhinosporidiosis

Rhinosporidiosis is a chronic granulomatous disease afflicting the mucosa of the nose, soft palate, and nasopharynx.

ETIOLOGY

Rhinosporidium seeberi is the suspected pathogen, although it has not been found in nature nor has it been grown in routine cultures. The infection occurs most commonly in the Indian subcontinent, with men working in agriculture being most often afflicted.

CLINICAL PRESENTATION

Sessile, friable, polypoid papules with whitish yellow dots resembling raspberries arise from the nasal mucosa, conjunctiva, tonsils, or larynx, and sometimes even the anal region. The lesions become pedunculated and protrude over the adjacent skin surface. They are often pruritic and associated with a mucoid discharge. Eventually, there is nasal obstruction (Figure 77).

DIAGNOSIS

Routine culturing may not be productive. Smears of the discharge stained with hematoxylin and eosin, periodic acid–Schiff, or Gomori stain often reveal the sporangia.

DIFFERENTIAL DIAGNOSIS

The lesions may be confused with other deep fungal infections, malignancy, granuloma inguinale, and pyogenic diseases.

TREATMENT

Wide excision or electrosurgery is used.

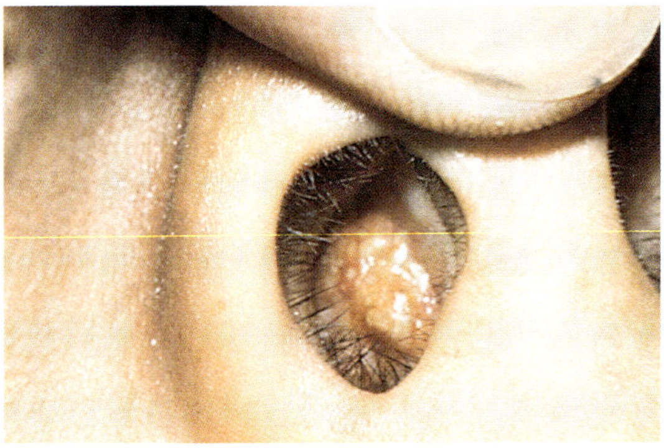

Figure 77
Rhinosporidiosis creates a granulomatous process in the nasal mucosa. (Courtesy of José Llevena, MD, El Salvador, San Salvador.)

SUGGESTED READINGS

Mahajan VM. Rhinosporidiosis. In: Mahgoub E-S, ed. Tropical mycoses. Beerse, Belgium: Janssen Research Council, 1991:175–184.

Yesudian P. Cutaneous rhinosporidiosis mimicking verruca vulgaris. Int J Dermatol 1988;27:47–48.

DIAGNOSIS

Culture of the organism or histologic examination will confirm the diagnosis. *H. capsulatum* var. *capsulatum* is very small and difficult to see on direct microscopy, whereas *H. capsulatum* var. *duboisii* forms larger yeasts in the tissue.

DIFFERENTIAL DIAGNOSIS

Lesions may resemble miliary tuberculosis, cryptococcosis, coccidioidomycosis, leishmaniasis, lymphomas, and even sarcoidosis.

TREATMENT

Itraconazole, 200 to 400 mg daily for an indefinite period, is recommended. Amphotericin B, 0.5 to 0.6 mg/kg IV, may be given daily during the acute stage and then weekly as a chronic suppressive regimen.

SUGGESTED READINGS

Drouhet E. Histoplasmosis. In: Mahgoub E-S, ed. Tropical Mycoses, Beerse, Belgium: Janssen Research Council, 1991:113–147.

Hay RJ. Histoplasmosis. Semin Dermatol 1993;12:310–314.

McKinsey DS, Smith DL, Driks MR, et al. Histoplasmosis in Missouri: historical review and current clinical concepts. Mo Med 1994;91:27–32.

Sharma OP. Histoplasmosis: a masquerader of sarcoidosis. Sarcoidosis 1991;8(1):10–13.

Swindells S, Dureham T, Johansson SL, et al. Oral histoplasmosis in a patient infected with HIV. A case report. Oral Surg Oral Med Oral Pathol 1994;77:126–130.

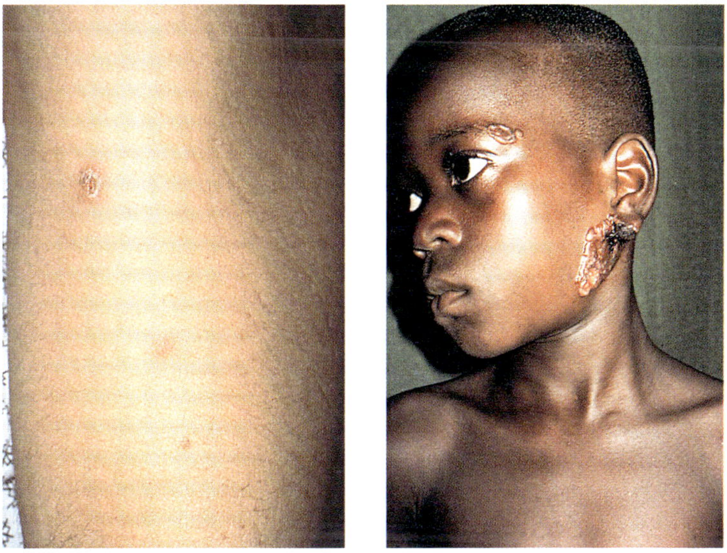

Figure 80
(a) Histoplasmosis may appear as erythematous papules, as seen in this AIDS patient. (Courtesy of Philip Cohen, MD, Houston, TX.) (b) African histoplasmosis represents a granulomatous process. (Courtesy of Wolfram Höffler, MD, Tübingen, Germany.)

a b

Coccidioidomycosis

Coccidioidomycosis is a systemic mycosis whose primary site of infection is usually the lungs.

ETIOLOGY

Coccidioides immitis is a dimorphous fungus found in nature and in cultures as a hyphal-arthrochondrial form, wheras in humans it is a spherule-endospore. The fungus has a propensity for semi-desert land with sandy soil, little rain, and high temperatures.

The disease it causes is endemic in the southwestern part of the United States, extending down through Mexico to parts of Central and South America. Non-Caucasians and immunosuppressed patients are more often afflicted, developing the symptoms in the dry season, which may extend from the late spring through the fall.

CLINICAL PRESENTATION

Following an incubation period of 1 to 4 weeks after inhalation of the spores, there may be an influenza-like illness or none at all. This primary infection may be accompanied by erythema nodosum, erythema multiforme, a papular urticaria, or a morbilliform eruption. As the disease becomes disseminated, there may be headache, bone pain, and specific cutaneous lesions. These lesions usually occur on the middle of the face or extremities, being characterized as papules, pustules, nodules, verrucous plaques, abscesses, draining sinuses, ulcers, cellulitis, and scars (Figure 81).

Rarely, there are primary cutaneous lesions. Such inoculation may appear as a nodule that ulcerates and then appears as a sporotrichoid lymphadenitis or regional lymphadenitis.

DIAGNOSIS

Clinical suspicion may be confirmed by culture and inoculation on laboratory animals. Special culturing techniques are needed to produce the endosporulating spherules. Skin biopsies, exudates, bronchial washings, and sputum may be stained with methenamine-silver or periodic acid–Schiff to highlight the organisms.

DIFFERENTIAL DIAGNOSIS

Many bacterial infections, such as folliculitis, furunculosis, or ecthyma, molluscum contagiosum, keratoacanthomas, tuberculosis, syphilis, and North American blastomycosis may look very much like this disease.

TREATMENT

Itraconazole, 100 mg bid, or amphotericin B, 0.5 to 0.6 mg/kg IV, is administered until the disease clears.

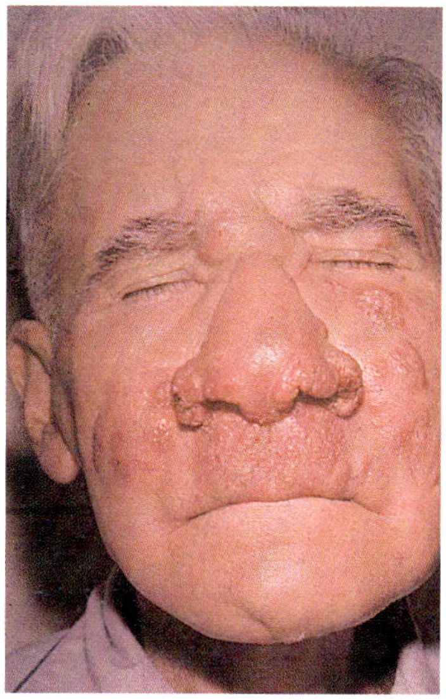

Figure 81
In coccidioidomycosis there are verrucous, scaling lesions on the face. (Courtesy of Ricardo Negroni, MD, Buenos Aries, Argentina.)

SUGGESTED READINGS

Galgiani JN. Coccidioidomycosis: changes in clinical expression, serological diagnosis, and therapeutic options. Clin Infect Dis 1992;14(suppl 1):S100–105.

Graybill JR. Treatment of coccidioidomycosis. Curr Top Med Mycol 1993;5:151–179.

Pappagianis D. Coccidioidomycosis. Semin Dermatol 1993;12:301–309.

Scully C, de Almeida OP. Orofacial manifestations of the systemic mycoses. J Oral Pathol Med 1992;21:289–294.

Sekhon AS, Isaac-Renton J, Dixon JM, et al. Review of human and animal cases of coccidioidomycosis diagnosed in Canada. Mycopathologia 1991;113:1–10.

Cryptococcosis

Cryptococcosis, also called *European blastomycosis*, is a pulmonary disease that is spread hematogenously. Primary cutaneous infection is rare.

ETIOLOGY

Cryptococcus neoformans exists in the yeast form in the environment, in infected tissue, and in cultures. The organism has been recovered worldwide from pigeon excreta, soil, and fruit. Cryptococcosis is more commonly found in men and patients with defective cellular immunity. Sarcoidosis and diabetes mellitus are other risk factors.

CLINICAL PRESENTATION

The initial pulmonary infection is usually asymptomatic. Dissemination to the meninges causes headaches, mental confusion, and facial neurologic signs. Cutaneous dissemination produces papules, pustules, nodules, abscesses, plaques, cellulitis, ulcers, and sinus tract formation. Lesions may occur anywhere but, most commonly, they occur on the face (Figure 82).

DIAGNOSIS

A skin biopsy will show encapsulated organisms that are best visualized by periodic acid –Schiff stain or methenamine–silver stain. Fungal cultures will also confirm the diagnosis. There is also a latex fixation test.

DIFFERENTIAL DIAGNOSIS

Many conditions, ranging from pyodermas and acne to herpes simplex infection, molluscum contagiosum, and basal cell cancer, may look like cryptococcosis.

TREATMENT

Combination therapy is most effective. Amphotericin B, 0.3 to 0.6 mg/kg/day IV, is combined with flucytosine, 150 mg/kg/day PO divided into four doses. Ketoconazole or fluconazole may provide an alternative.

SUGGESTED READINGS

Berger TG. Treatment of bacterial, fungal, and parasitic infections in the HIV-infected host. Semin Dermatol 1993;12:296–300.

Chick SL, Sande MA. Infections with *Cryptococcus neoformans* in the acquired immunodeficiency syndrome. N Engl J Med 1989;321:794–932.

Durden FA, Elewski B. Cutaneous involvement with *Cryptococcus neoformans* in AIDS. J Am Acad Dermatol 1994;30:844–848.

Kappe R, Seeliger H. Serodiagnosis of deep-seated fungal infections. Curr Top Med Mycol 1993;5:247–280.

Ng WF, Loo KT. Cutaneous cryptococcosis—primary versus secondary disease. Am J Dermatopathol 1993;15:372–377.

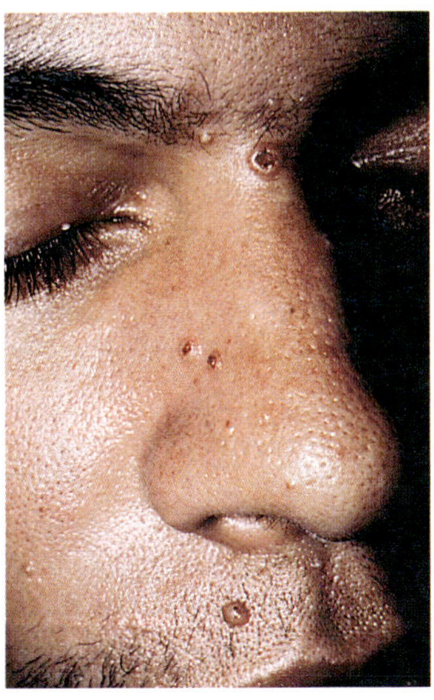

Figure 82
Cryptococcosis may appear as molluscum-like lesions, as shown on the face of this AIDS patient. (Courtesy of Sebastião AP Sampãio, MD, São Paulo, Brazil.)

Actinomycosis

Actinomycosis is caused by an anaerobic gram-positive bacterium, but it is grouped with the deep fungal infections due to convention and its clinical presentations.

ETIOLOGY

The disease is most often caused by *Actinomyces israelii*. Other organisms sometimes responsible are *A. bovis*, *A. naeslundii*, and *A. viscosus*. A. bovis has never been isolated outside the human body, where it may be found in the mouth, tonsils, or carious teeth. Actinomycosis is acquired by endogenous implantation into tissue where anaerobic conditions are present. Some of the routes of infection are dental extractions, puncture wounds, and inhalation.

CLINICAL PRESENTATION

While the disease may occur on an extremity following a compound fracture, it is most often seen on the face, abdomen, or thorax. The initial manifestation is dusky, red, nontender, firm nodules. Each becomes fluctuant and breaks down to form sinuses, draining pus with whitish or yellowish granules. The entire area is surrounded by "wooden" induration, producing a "lumpy jaw" in the cervicofacial area (Figure 83). In abdominal actinomycosis, there may be underlying diseases of the cecum, stomach, gallbladder, urinary bladder, or genitalia. With bone involvement, there may be preexisting periostitis or osteomyelitis.

DIAGNOSIS

Pus or biopsy specimens should be examined for sulfur granules. Gram stain of a crushed granule will show delicately branching gram-positive filaments. Culture of a granule on brain-heart infusion agar at 37°C under anaerobic conditions will produce growth.

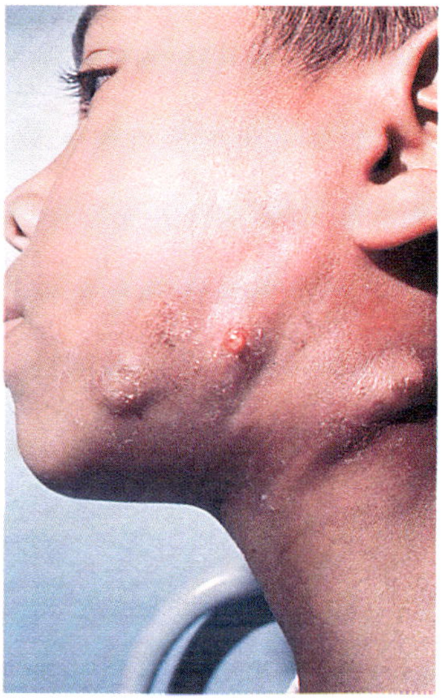

Figure 83
The lumpy nodules characteristic of actinomycosis are often found on the jaw. (Courtesy of Antar Padilha-Gonçalves, MD, Rio de Janeiro, Brazil.)

DIFFERENTIAL DIAGNOSIS

Actinomycosis may appear similar to scrofuloderma, North American blastomycosis, tertiary syphilis, or various sarcomas.

TREATMENT

Penicillin, 10 to 20 million units IV daily for a month, followed by penicillin, 4 to 6 gm PO for 2 months is often recommended. Sulfonamides and quinolones should also be effective. Sometimes surgical incision, drainage, and debridement are needed.

SUGGESTED READINGS

Foster SV, Demmier GJ, Hawkins EP, et al. Pediatric cervicofacial actinomycosis. South Med J 1993;86:1147–1150.

Kawai M, Mizutani H, Ueda M, et al. Cervicofacial actinomycosis: report of two cases. Nagoya J Med Sci 1993;55:83–88.

Paulker SG, Kopelman RI. Clinical problem-solving. A rewarding pursuit of certainty. N Engl J Med 1993;329:1103–1107.

PARASITES

Parasites are those organisms that have adapted to life by living in the tissue of the host, as opposed to saprophytes, which do not require a living host. Commensals do not cause disease, although they live both inside and on the surface of the host.

Animal parasites that afflict humans belong to three phyla: Protozoa (unicellular), Helminthes (worms), and Arthropoda (invertebrates). They may be classified as ectoparasites (i.e., adapted to existence on the skin surface) and endoparasites (which live inside the human body). Practically all kinds of parasites may cause skin changes, ranging from simple itching to a well-characterized disease.

SUPERFICIAL PARASITIC INFESTATIONS

Ectoparasites are mainly arthropods. Two classes of great importance are Arachnida (spiders, scorpions, ticks, and mites) and Insecta (lice, bedbugs, and fleas). They produce parasitic disease, either by living permanently on the skin, as in the scabies mite, or by a transient contact for feeding, as in lice. In both cases, irritative or allergic reactions occur in the human host. The pruritus often created may lead to secondary bacterial infection. So-called innocent insect bites may actually foretell more serious bacterial, rickettsial, viral, or parasitic diseases.

SCABIES

Scabies, the so called seven-year itch, can create one of the most severe pruritic states known to humans.

ETIOLOGY

The *Sarcoptes scabiei* var. *hominis* is hardly perceptible to the naked eye. It measures 270 to 380 μm, while the ova are 100 × 150 μm. The fertile female mite burrows into the keratin layer to lay her eggs, giving rise to adult mites in 10 to 14 days. The life cycle is 30 days. Transmission is due to direct skin-to-skin contact in almost all instances.

CLINICAL PRESENTATION

A patient who presents with itching approaching 100% on a 1 to 100 grading scale has scabies until proved otherwise. This is due to the movement of the female mite. The characteristic burrow, being a 2- to 4-mm uneven line with a vesicle at one end, may not be visualized; however, the red urticarial papules or inflammatory vesicles will be found predominantly in the finger webs (Figure 84a), areas of pressure such as under a bra or a belt, and on the genitalia (Figure 84b). Although the scabies mite prefers warmth, areas such as the axilla or the inguinal region are too hot. The face is spared, except in children and in immunocompromised patients. Crusts and excoriations are seen on the trunk and extremities.

Elderly patients may present with a nonspecific dermatitis that resembles neurodermatitis (Figure 84c), while other patients may simply have a few excoriations. *Crusted scabies*, improperly termed *Norwegian scabies*, occurs in immunocompromised patients (Figure 84d).

DIAGNOSIS

A scraping of a pruritic papule or burrow, preferably not an excoriated one, will reveal under microscopic examination the mite, eggs, or fecal pellets.

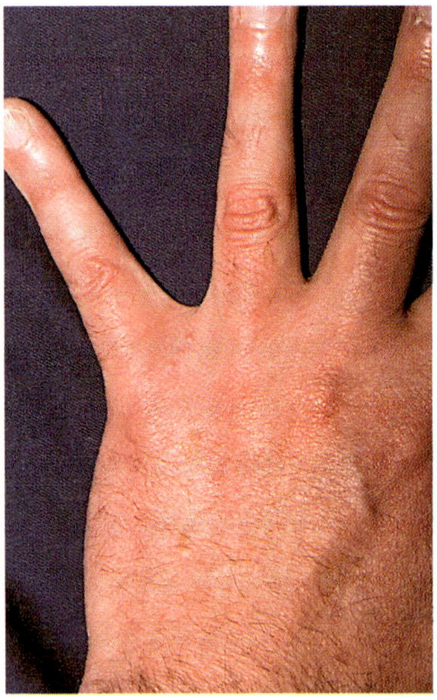

a

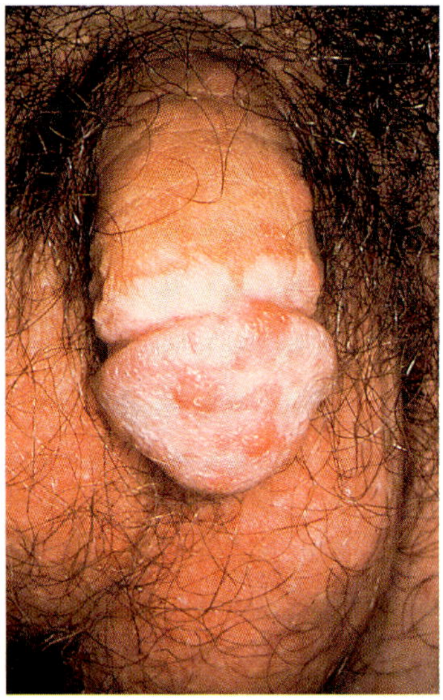

b

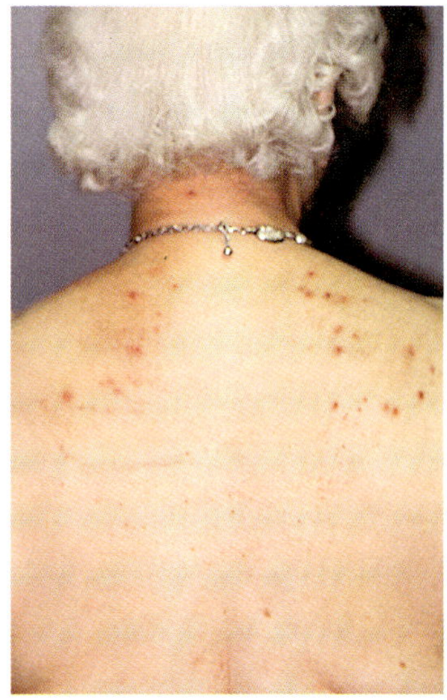

c

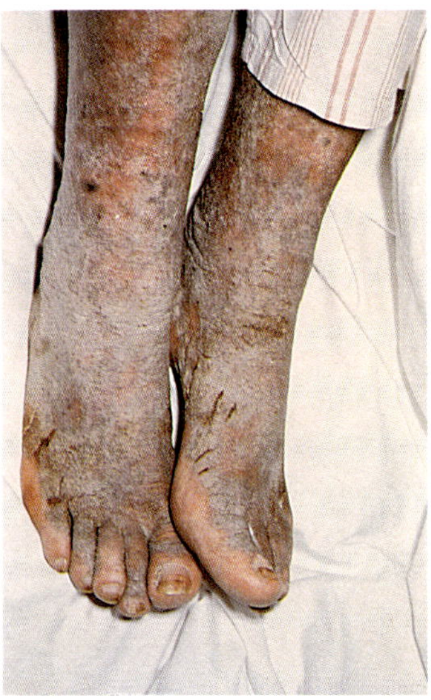

d

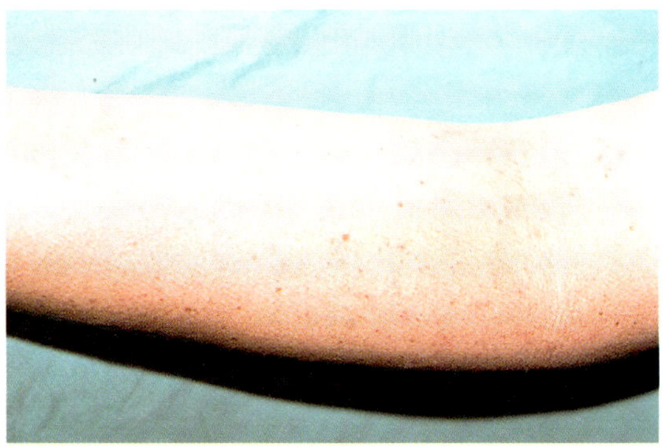

e

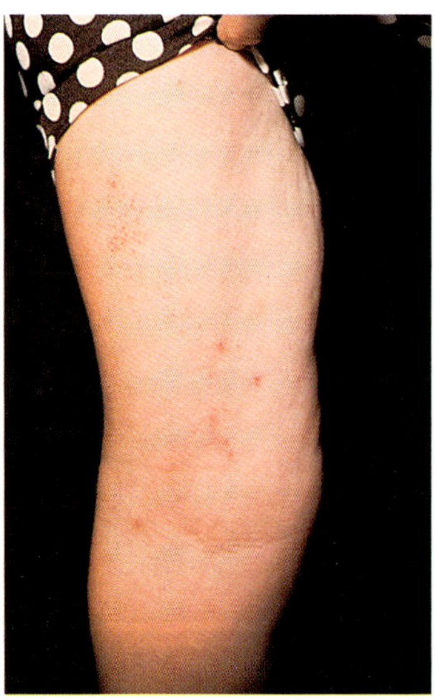

f

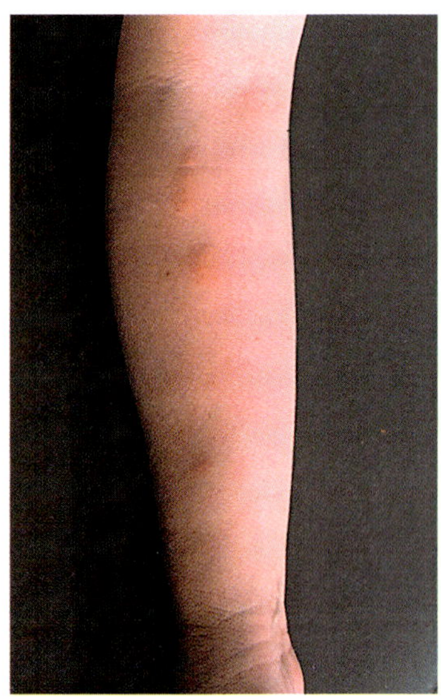

g

DIFFERENTIAL DIAGNOSIS

Scabies can be confused with contact dermatitis, neurodermatitis, and even a drug eruption. The canine scabies mite causes a morbilliform eruption in the areas where the infested dog is hugged (Figure 84e). A similar eruption is caused by *Cheyletiella*, a mite found predominantly in rabbits and cats (Figure 84f). Another mite, *Dermanyssus gallinae* (red poultry mite), causes red urticarial lesions (Figure 84g) that can be confused with scabies.

TREATMENT

Lindane 1% lotion or permethrin 5% cream, applied from the neck to the toes for 12 hours, will kill the mite. There is no known resistance to treatment from these preparations; rather, the patient may not have applied the medicament under the nails or there was reinfestation from a partner. Benzyl benzoate emulsion is the preferred agent in many parts of Europe. An alternative for patients not wishing chemicals applied to their skin is an ointment of 6% precipitated sulfur applied daily for 3 days. Contacts and household members should also be treated. In immune depressed patients, the face should be treated and a second application of the medicament applied in 3 to 7 days.

SUGGESTED READINGS

Alexander JO. Arthropods and human skin. New York: Springer-Verlag, 1985:115–208.

Angarano DW, Parish LC. Comparative dermatology: parasitic disorders. Clin Dermatol 1994;12:543–550.

Burgess I. *Sarcoptes scabiei* and scabies. Adv Parasitol 1994;33:235–292.

Parish LC, Nutting WB, Schwartzman RM. Cutaneous infestations of man and animal. New York: Praeger Scientific, 1983:53–106.

Parish LC, Schwartzman RM. Zoonoses of dermatological interest. Semin Dermatol 1993;12:57–64.

Parish LC, Witkowski JA. Scabies and pediculosis. In: Parish LC, Gschnait F, eds. Sexually transmitted diseases: a guide for clinicians. New York: Springer-Verlag, 1989:157–165.

Parish LC, Witkowski JA, Millikan LE. Scabies in the extended care facility. Int J Dermatol 1991;30:703–706.

Figure 84
Scabies characteristically has red papules (a) in the finger webs and (b) on the penis. (c) Older patients may have nonspecific lesions on the trunk that are easily confused with those of neurodermatitis. (d) Crusted scabies can cover large areas with huge numbers of mites. (e) Dogs who are infested with *Sarcoptes scabiei* var. *canis* may create a red papular eruption at the site on humans where they are held. (f) Infestations with the *Chyletiella* species are characterized by a red, almost nondescript, eruption on the flanks. (Courtesy of Peter J Ihrke, VMD, Davis, CA.) (g) *Dermanyssus gallinae* (red poultry mite) created red, urticarial lesions in this physician who was vacationing on the Amalfi Coast. In this patient, pigeons were the vectors.

Pediculosis

Pediculosis may be divided into three conditions in humans: pediculosis capitis, pediculosis corporis, and phthiriasis pubis. The causative agents are blood-sucking insects from the family Pediculidae and the order Anoplura.

ETIOLOGY

The head louse, *Pediculus capitis*, differs from the body louse, *Pediculus corporis*, by being 2 to 4 mm long as opposed to 3 to 4.5 mm. Both have three pairs of legs, and the female lays up to 300 eggs (0.8 to 1 mm) or nits during her approximate 30-day life cycle. The louse pierces the skin every few hours for a blood meal and can live away from the host for about 2 days.

The crab louse, *Pthirus pubis*, has legs that resemble those of crabs. It measures 1.5 mm in length and has a different appearance.

CLINICAL PRESENTATION

The head louse is found in preadolescent children and almost never in African-American patients. It lives on the scalp hair, where nits can be found. It can cause itching of the scalp so that excoriations are sometimes seen on the neck (Figure 85a).

The body louse stays in the seams of clothing, piercing the skin for a blood meal. This results in extensive pruritus on the body, sometimes called *vagabond's disease* (Figure 85b). Only the body louse is a vector for other diseases including epidemic typhus (*Rickettsia prowazekii*), trench fever (*Rickettsia quintana*), and relapsing fever (*Borrelia recurrentis*).

The pubic louse is not only found on the pubic hair but also anywhere else on the body where there is hair. The points of biting may turn a slate gray, maculae cerulea (0.5 × 0.5 mm). When found on the eyelashes, the condition is termed *pediculosis ciliaris* (Figure 85c).

DIAGNOSIS

Finding the louse on the hair or on the clothing will confirm the diagnosis. Living nits, being whitish, are attached to the hairs or clothing fibers.

DIFFERENTIAL DIAGNOSIS

Seborrheic dermatitis, contact dermatitis, and possibly a drug eruption might be confused with pediculosis.

TREATMENT

Shampooing with lindane 1% shampoo for 4 minutes and repeating in 7 days should alleviate pediculosis capitis and pediculosis pubis. Pemethrin 5% cream or shampoo or copper oleate cream may also be used. Contacts and household members should be treated as well.

For pediculosis corporis, fumigating or destroying the clothes is all that is required. Symptomatic topical therapy may be used in addition.

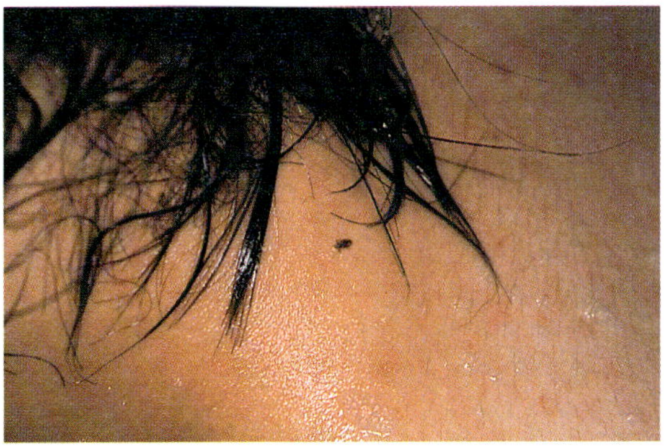

a

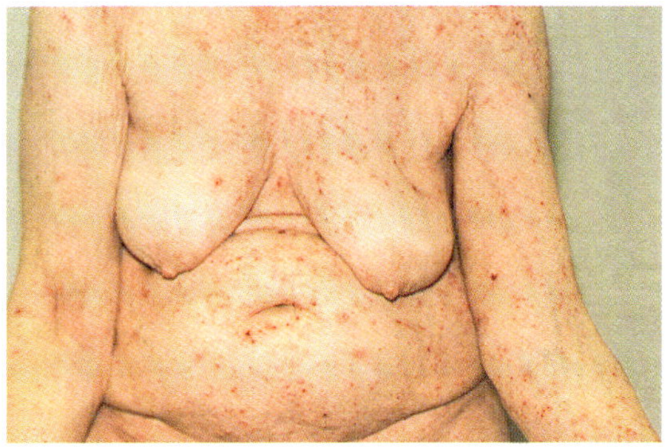

b

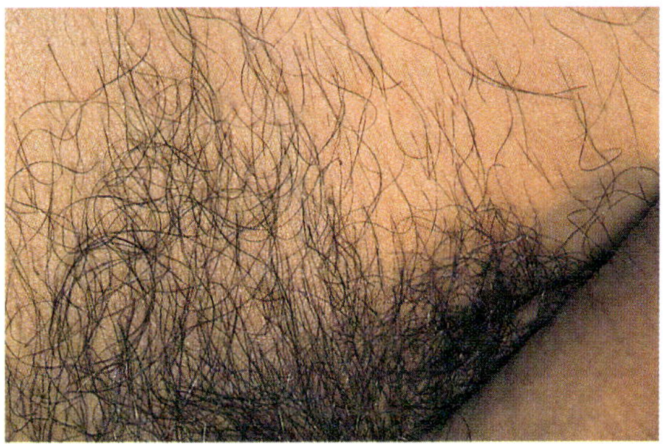

c

Figure 85
(a) Pediculosis capitis may be identified by nits on the hair and is characterized by dermatitis on the neck. A louse is present on the skin. (b) Pediculosis corporis shows diffuse excoriations and often linear scratch marks. (c) Phthiriasis pubis demonstrates subtle puncture wounds on the skin. Observing the live louse is often difficult without manifestations.

SUGGESTED READINGS

Alexander JO. Arthropods and human skin. New York: Springer-Verlag, 1985:29–55.

Parish LC, Nutting WB, Schwartzman RM. Cutaneous infestations of man and animal. New York: Praeger Scientific, 1983:113–180.

Parish LC, Witkowski JA. Scabies and pediculosis. In: Parish LC, Gschnait F, eds. Sexually transmitted diseases: a guide for clinicians. New York: Springer-Verlag, 1989:157–165.

Sholt LL, Holloway ML, Fronk WD. The epidemiology of human pediculosis in Ethiopia. Jacksonville, FL: Navy Disease Vector Ecology and Control Center, 1979:1–150.

Sundnes KO, Haimanot AT. Epidemic of louse-borne relapsing fever in Ethiopia. Lancet 1993;343:1213–1215.

Bedbug Bites

Bedbug bites (cimicidosis) create unpleasant bites in the strangest places. These insects have periodically been thought to carry disease, including hepatitis B, but confirmation has not been forthcoming.

ETIOLOGY

Cimex is a member of the Cimicidae family, Hemiptera order. Two types are known: *C. lectularius*, the common bedbug, and *C. tropica*, the tropical bedbug. *C. lectularius* measures 3 to 6 mm, is brownish, six-legged, flat, and oval. The bedbug feeds at night and can live for up to a year without a meal, having a life cycle of 6 to 8 months. It prefers dark places such as furniture cracks or under the mattress buttons.

CLINICAL PRESENTATION

The bite is usually painless, and the site becomes a pruritic wheal with a hemorrhagic center (Figure 86). The lesion may become bullous and emits a characteristic odor. Bites are found more often on the face, neck, arms, and hands. The number of bites may vary and the so-called traditional row of three may be a single bite or many.

DIAGNOSIS

Finding the bedbug in the bed or in the room suggests the diagnosis.

DIFFERENTIAL DIAGNOSIS

Bedbug bites can resemble other insect bites, particularly when they have become eczematized. The bites may resemble urticaria, bullous pemphigoid, and even drug eruptions.

TREATMENT

Bedbugs are easily destroyed by such insecticides as pyrethrins and malathion.

SUGGESTED READINGS

Alexander JO. Arthropods and human skin. New York: Springer-Verlag, 1985:57–74.

The bed-bug. London: Trustees of the British Museum (Natural History), 1977:1–17.

Crissey JT. Bedbugs: an old problem with a new dimension. Int J Dermatol 1981;20:411–414.

Fletcher MG, Axtell RC. Susceptibility of the bedbug, *Cimex lectularius*, to selected insecticides and various treated surfaces. Med Vet Entomol 1993;7:69–72.

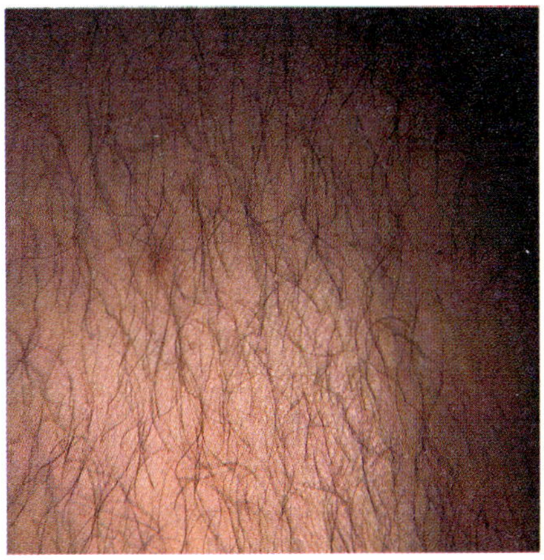

Figure 86
Bedbug bites present as red papules, not always in groups of three.

Flea Bites

Flea bites, also known as *pulicosis*, afflict humans and their pets, particularly dogs and cats.

ETIOLOGY

Humans currently are afflicted more often by the cat flea (*Ctenocephalides felis*) and less frequently by the human flea (*Pulex irritans*) or the dog flea (*Ctenocephalides canis*). Fleas are small (1 to 2 mm) actively jumping, blood-sucking insects from the family Pulicidae, order Siphonaptera. They hide in cracks in the floor, crevices in upholstered furniture, areas under carpets, and parts of the bed or pet baskets. Fleas tend to bite at night. Although fleas prefer animals for a blood meal, they resort to humans when the pet is no longer present. The adult female has a life span of 6 to 12 months and lays as many as 20 to 25 eggs per day.

CLINICAL PRESENTATION

Flea bites occur on uncovered parts of the body, especially on the legs. Fresh lesions are often groups and represent intensely pruritic wheals with central hemorrhagic puncta. These lesions quickly resolve, leaving small, dark red, excoriated papules. *Purpura pulicosa* refers to a marked hemorrhagic eruption, occurring in sensitized patients (Figure 87a,b).

Tungiasis, or chigoe (chigger) bites, represent a special form of flea bite caused by the sand flea *Tunga penetrans*, encountered in the tropics or subtropics. The female burrows into the soft skin of the feet, particularly between the toes and nail folds, resulting in itching, inflammation, secondary infection, and even abscess formation (Figure 87c).

DIAGNOSIS

The clinical symptoms and history of contact with cats and dogs suggest the diagnosis.

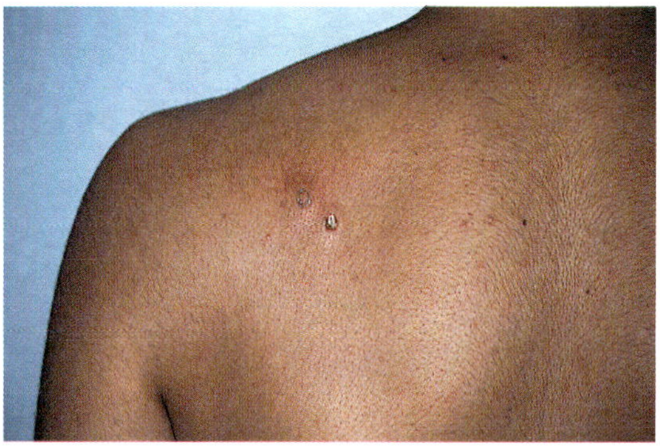

a

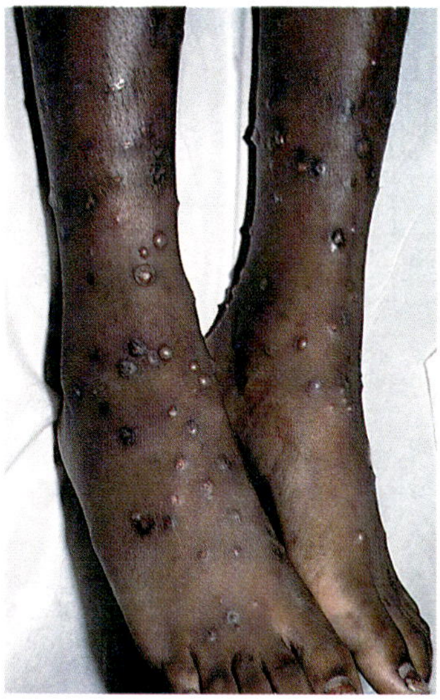

b

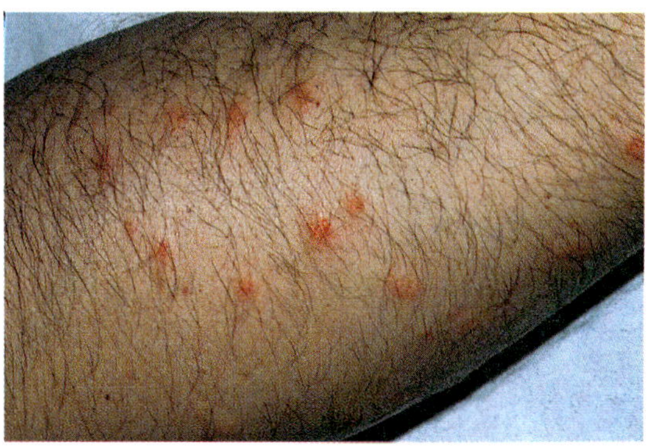

c

Figure 87
Flea bites can appear (a) as innocuous papules on the back or (b) as papules, vesicles, and crusted lesions on the legs. (c) Tungiasis is known by the intensely red papules produced.

DIFFERENTIAL DIAGNOSIS

Other insect bites and resulting papular urticaria can mimic flea bites. An excellent clue for the diagnosis of flea bites is learning of the departure of a pet from the house or environs, leaving newly hatched fleas searching for a blood meal.

TREATMENT

Elimination of the fleas from the pet is the key. This involves insecticidal dips. Houses and particularly rugs and upholstered furniture need fumigation. Patients are treated symptomatically with topical steroids.

SUGGESTED READINGS

Angarano DW, Parish LC. Comparative dermatology: parasitic disorders. Clin Dermatol 1994;12:543–550.

Fichter GS. Insect pests. New York: Golden Press, 1966:1–160.

Kauh YC, Ruschak PJ, Luscombe HA. Histopathologic manifestations of cutaneous arthropod infestations. In: Parish LC, Nutting WB, Schwartzman RM, eds. Cutaneous infestations of man and animal. New York: Praeger Scientific, 1983:25–42.

Medleau L, Miller WH. Flea infestation and its control. Int J Dermatol 1983;22:378–379.

Parish LC, Schwartzman RM. Zoonoses of dermatological interest. Semin Dermatol 1993;12:57–64.

Smith FGAM. Siphonaptera (fleas). In: Smith KGV, ed. Insect and other arthropods of medical importance. London: Trustees of the British Museum, 1973:325–371.

Tick Bites

Tick bites are usually harmless; however, the fact that they are vectors for Lyme borreliosis, Rocky Mountain spotted fever, tick-born relapsing fever, and tularemia make them a concern of the public.

ETIOLOGY

Ticks (order Acarina) are blood-sucking ectoparasites of wild and domestic animals, rodents, and humans. Two families of ticks exist: the hard ticks (Ixodidae) living in wooded areas worldwide, and the soft ticks (Argasidae) found in the tropics and subtropics, which are only slightly less hard than the Ixodidae. Ticks feed by inserting their mouthparts into the host's skin, remaining there for several days until fully engorged with blood.

CLINICAL PRESENTATION

Ticks have a predilection for biting near skin folds. The bites of the hard tick usually remain unnoticed as an anesthetic and anticoagulant substance is introduced. The bite of the soft tick may be more painful. Sometimes, mild pruritus and surrounding erythema occur. When the area is scratched or the tick is forcefully removed, mouth parts may remain, which lead to possible pyoderma or granuloma formation (Figure 88).

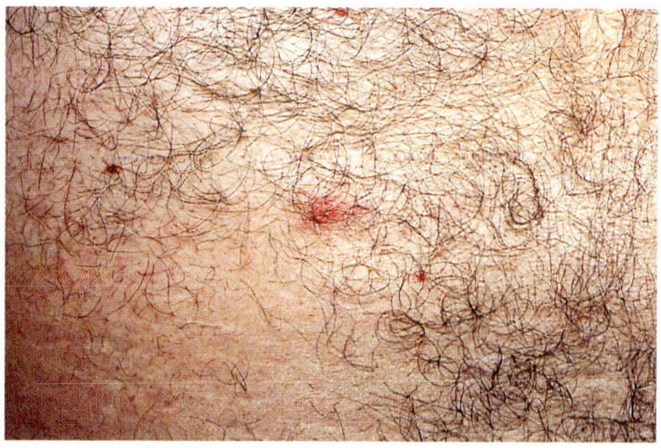

Figure 88
Tick bites often develop into inflammatory nodules.

DIAGNOSIS

Finding the tick or its parts still attached suggests the diagnosis.

DIFFERENTIAL DIAGNOSIS

Other insect bites will look very similar.

TREATMENT

The tick may be covered with oil. In a few minutes, it should drop off. Skeletal parts should be picked off of the host.

SUGGESTED READINGS

Cupp EW. Biology of ticks. Vet Clin North Am Small Animal Pract 1991;21:1–26.

Krinsky WL. Dermatoses associated with the bites of mites and ticks (Arthropoda: Acari). Int J Dermatol 1983;22:75–91.

Spach DH, Liles WC, Campbell GR, et al. Tick-borne diseases in the United States. N Engl J Med 1993;329:936–947.

Fly Bites and Myiasis

Fly bites and myiasis result from piercing of the skin or from larvae found on or in the skin.

ETIOLOGY

There are over 100 species of flies involved, ranging from *Lucullia illustris* (the blue-bottle fly) to the Tabanus species (horseflies). The adult fly bites the skin, whereas the larvae feed on or in the skin or wound.

CLINICAL PRESENTATION

Fly bites may be simply bite marks or urticarial lesions. The larvae may erode a wound or create a nodule under the skin (Figure 89a,b).

DIAGNOSIS

Observing the insects will confirm the diagnosis.

DIFFERENTIAL DIAGNOSIS

Other insect bites, creeping eruptions, or foreign bodies may be confused with this condition.

TREATMENT

Bites are treated symptomatically with topical steroids. Myiasis may require surgical excision. Sometimes placing meat on the surface of the lesion will bring the larvae out of the wound.

SUGGESTED READINGS

Allen JR. Mosquitoes and other biting flies. In: Parish LC, Nutting WB, Schwartzman RM, eds. Cutaneous infestations of man and animal. New York: Praeger Scientific, 1983:344–354.

Borror DJ, White RE. A field guide to insects: America north of Mexico. Boston: Houghton Mifflin, 1970:1–404.

Davies M, Kathirithamby J. Greek insects. Oxford: Oxford University Press, 1986:1–211.

Liu H, Buck HW. Cutaneous myiasis: a simple and effective technique for extraction of *Dermatoiba hominis* larvae. Int J Dermatol 1992;31:657–659.

Noutsis C, Millikan LE. Myiasis. Dermatol Clin 1994;12:729–736.

Nutting WB, Parish LC. Larval invasions. In: Parish LC, Nutting WB, Schwartzman RM, eds. Cutaneous infestations of man and animal. New York: Praeger Scientific, 1983:356–359.

Pampiglione S, Bettoli V, Cestari G, et al. Miasi da *Cordylobia anthropophaga*: 7 casi su turisti italiani di ritorno dal Senegal. Ann Ital Dermatol Clin Sper 1993;47:195–200.

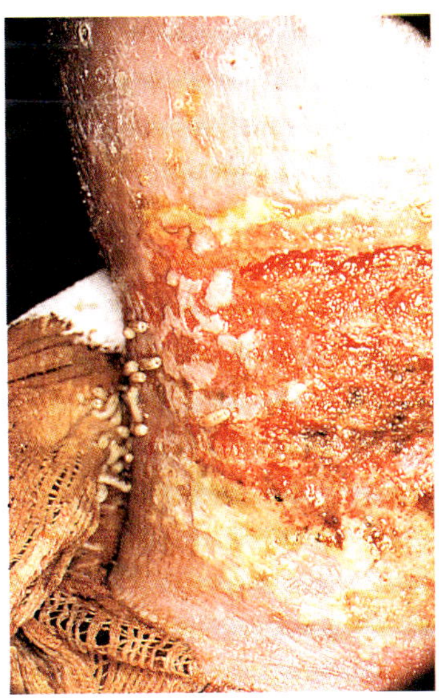

a

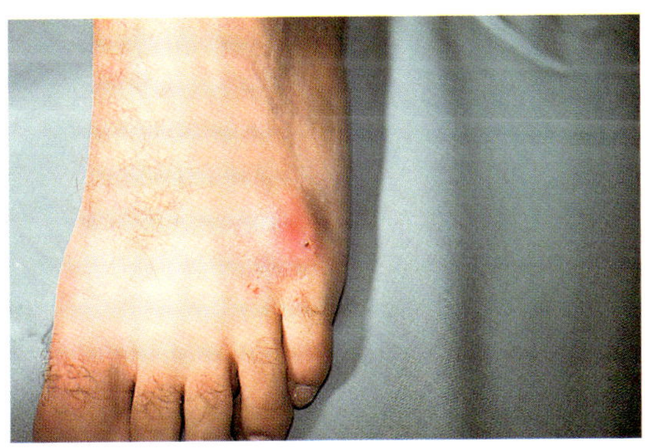

b

Figure 89
(a) Maggots are sometimes found in open ulcers, particularly when the hygiene has not been good. (b) Myiasis may appear as draining nodules containing the larvae. (Courtesy of Harvey Lui, MD, Vancouver, BC, Canada. Reproduced by permission from Int J Dermatol 1992;31:657–659.)

Arachnidism

Arachnidism or spider bites can cause severe cutaneous and systemic reactions.

ETIOLOGY

Spiders (order Aracneida) are carnivorous eight-legged arachnids that capture their prey, usually arthropods, by injecting a neurotoxic venom. From the numerous species encountered worldwide, only a few may be dangerous to humans. These include the black widow spider, *Lactrodectus mactans*, and the brown recluse spider, *Loxosceles reclusa*, both found in North America. *L. reclusa* is found in South America as well. European species seem to cause little or no harm.

CLINICAL PRESENTATION

Lactodelism, the black widow spider bite, is marked by sharp but short local pain and a lack of cutaneous changes. Within 15 minutes, systemic neurotoxic effects appear, including chills, headache, hypertension, mental changes (anxiety, manic, confusion), generalized muscle cramps, tremor, rigidity (especially abdominal), and paralysis. Symptoms usually resolve within 2 days, but rarely in young children and the infirm, central nervous system effects may be severe enough to be lethal (Figure 90a).

Loxoscelism, the brown recluse spider bite, causes two types of reactions: dermonecrosis (sphingomyelinase D), with local pain, ischemia, and necrosis with slowly healing ulcerations, and systemic reactions, including intoxication, hemolysis, hematuria, thrombocytopenia, sometimes renal failure, and even disseminated intravascular coagulopathy (Figure 90b).

DIAGNOSIS

Knowing the environment and suspecting a spider bite will assist in making the diagnosis. The black widow spider has an hourglass-like marking on the abdomen, and the brown recluse spider has a violin-like marking on the back.

DIFFERENTIAL DIAGNOSIS

A neurotizing infection such as necrotizing fasciitis may resemble reactions to spider bites. A drug reaction or infected foreign-body reaction could also have similar presentations.

TREATMENT

Most often, cleaning the bite and applying cold compresses is sufficient. However, for severe lactodelism, muscle relaxants and specific equine antivenom are necessary. With *Loxosceles*, avoiding surgery and use of either steroids or dapsone are recommended.

SUGGESTED READINGS

Alexander JO. Arthropods and human skin. New York: Springer-Verlag, 1985:209–226.

Alexander PC. Loxoscelism and the history of the Missouri brown spider: recollection of Dr. Joseph Flynn. Mo Med 1990;87:747–752.

King LE. Spider bites. Arch Dermatol 1987;123:41–43.

Millikan LE. Loxoscelism and other arachnid problems. In: Parish LC, Nutting WB, Schwartzman RM, eds. Cutaneous infestations of man and animal. New York: Praeger Scientific, 1983:284–295.

Reisman RE. Insect stings. N Engl J Med 1994;331:523–527.

Figure 90
(a) In lactodelism, there is a punctate wound with surrounding erythema and induration. (b) In loxoscelism, there is severe necrosis and destruction of tissue. (Courtesy of Philip Anderson, MD, Columbia, MO.)

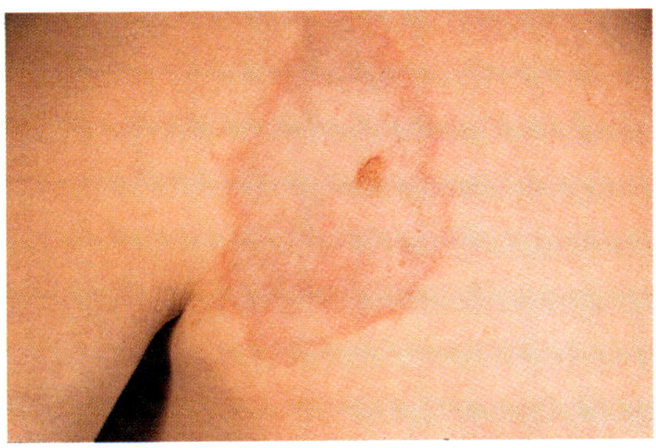

a

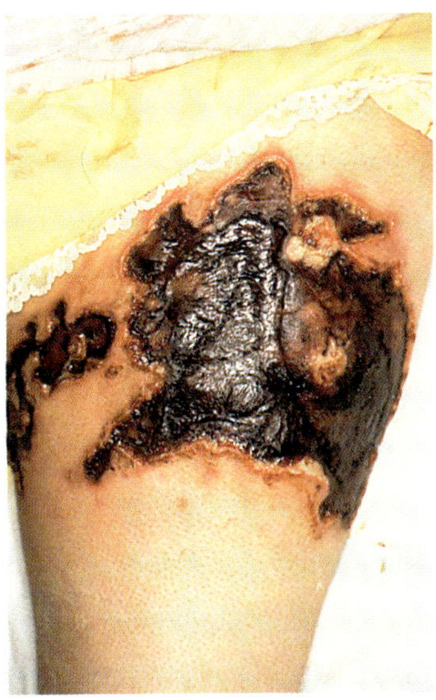

b

DEEP PARASITIC INFESTATIONS

Endoparasites, as the name implies, live within the body, attacking visceral organs and using the hematologic system for transportation. They are protozoa and worms, the latter being round worms (Nemathelminthes) and flat worms (Plathelminthes). Endoparasites are often transmitted to humans by arthropod vectors. Other hosts such as wild and domestic animals serve as the natural reservoir in the endemic areas.

LEISHMANIASIS

Leishmaniasis is a chronic granulomatous protozoan infection. It can be divided into *kala-azar*, or visceral leishmaniasis, and *cutaneous leishmaniasis*.

ETIOLOGY

Leishmaniae are flagellate protozoa that invade the cells of the mononuclear phagocytic system. Over 200 species are known. Of significance to the dermatologist are *Leishmania donovani*, the cause of kala-azar, *L. tropica*, the cause of cutaneous leishmaniasis, and *L. braziliensis*, the cause of American mucocutaneous leishmaniasis. The endemic areas are the tropics and subtropics, where the parasites are transmitted by the bites of sandflies, belonging to the genera Phlebotomus and Lutzomyia. Leishmanial infections induce cell-mediated immune responses.

Table 12 Cutaneous Involvement in Leishmaniasis

Species	Clinical form	Pathogenesis
visceral—*L. donovani*	kala-azar	nonspecific
	post-Kala-azar dermal leishmanid	hematogenous
cutaneous—*L. tropica*	oriental sore	inoculation
	leishmaniasis recidivans	id reaction
muco-cutaneous—*L. braziliensis*	cutaneous American leishmaniasis	inoculation
	mucocutaneous American leishmaniasis	hematogenous, lymphatogenous
	disseminated American leishmaniasis	hematogenous, lymphatogenous

CLINICAL PRESENTATION

Cutaneous involvement may be classified according to the implicated species, the type of the skin reaction, and the immune competence of the individual (Table 12). The skin lesions are the prototype of delayed skin hypersensitivity to the leishmanial antigens.

Kala-azar, or visceral leishmaniasis Characterized by fever, anemia, hepatomegaly, splenomegaly, and lymphadenopathy. The skin changes, characteristic for the active stage, are generalized earth-gray hyperpigmentation and atrophy.

Post-kala-azar dermal leishmaniasis Occurs in the chronic stage. Hypochromic macules, facial heliotropic erythema, and disseminated soft nodules of different sizes are the typical lesions (Figure 91a).

Localized cutaneous leishmaniasis or oriental sore Occurs at the site of the sandfly bite, usually the face, arms, and legs. The incubation period is 2 to 3 weeks and up to several months. The primary lesion is an erythematous infiltrated papule with raised borders that ulcerate in the center. Spontaneous healing takes up to a year, leaving a disfiguring scar. Permanent immunity is usually acquired (Figure 91b,c).

Leishmaniasis recidivans Characterized by the appearance of satellite lesions at the periphery or at some distance from a preexisting scar of an Oriental sore. The lesions represent tuberculoid papules and nodules, forming circinate, peripherally active plaques with central healing (Figure 91d).

Cutaneous American leishmaniasis, or uta Resembles Oriental sore in the primary stage. It later differs by having more pronounced ulceration, impetigination, and regional lymphadenopathy. There is no permanent immunity (Figure 91e).

Mucocutaneous American leishmaniasis, or espundia Develops several years after the healing of the primary lesions. The cutaneous lesions may be ulcerated, vegetative, or sporotrichoid. Mucous membrane lesions affect mainly the upper lip and nasal septum, resulting in severe mutilation. There may be progressive involvement of the pharynx, larynx, trachea, and lung (Figure 91f,g).

Disseminated American leishmaniasis Characterized by an anergic state and disseminated persistent lepromata-like lesions, rich in parasites. Highly malignant in its progression, the disease responds poorly to treatment and rarely regresses (Figure 91h).

Figure 91
Leishmaniasis takes many forms. (a) Post-kala-azar dermal leishmaniasis is characterized by red to purplish lesions. (Courtesy of Patrick Yesudian, MD, Madras, India.) (b) The Oriental sore appears as an ulcer with heaped-up borders. (c) Cutaneous leishmaniasis usually develops as a crusted lesion at the site of the sandfly bites. (Courtesy of Wolfram Höffler, MD, Tübingen, Germany.) (d) Leishman-iasis recidivans appears as a large plaque with heaped-up borders. (e) Cutaneous American leishmaniasis also begins with crusted lesions. (Courtesy of Wolfram Höffler, MD, Tübingen, Germany.) The mucocutaneous form can show (f) redness and erosions in the mouth. (g) The mucocutaneous form can also progress to massive destruction as an espundia necrotizing granuloma. (h) Anergic leishmaniasis may present with a nonspecific erythematous eruption.

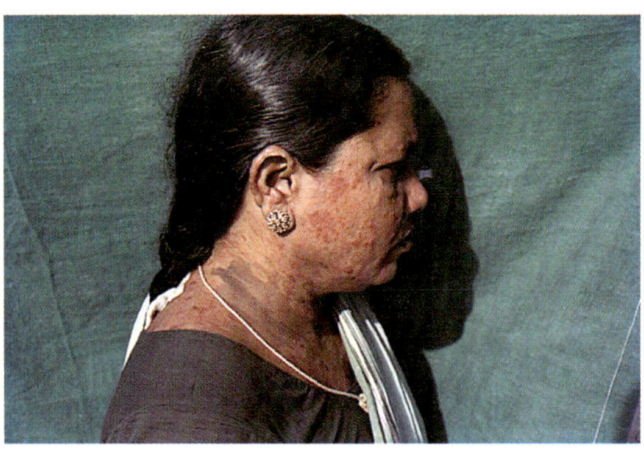

a

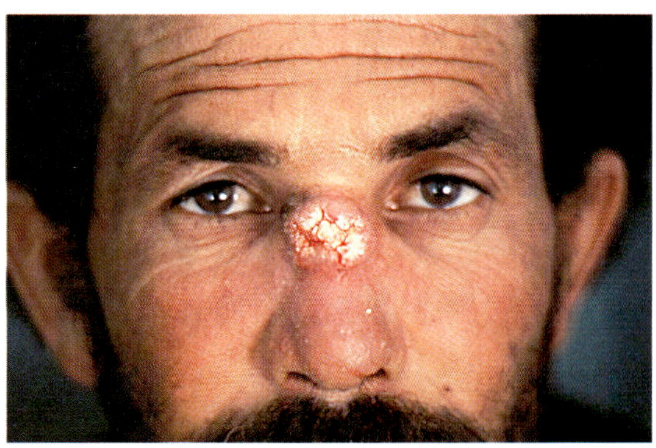

b

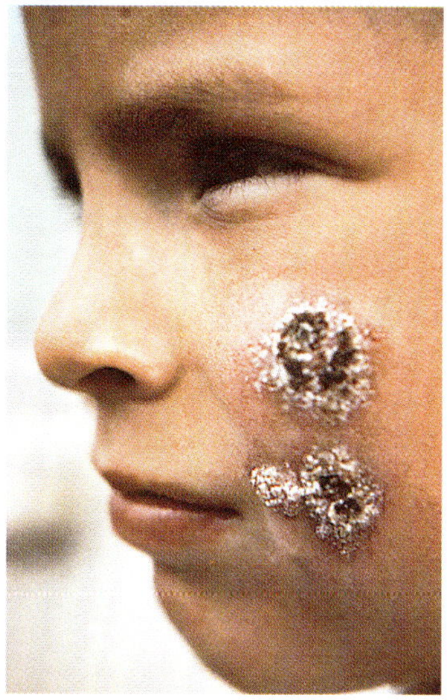

c

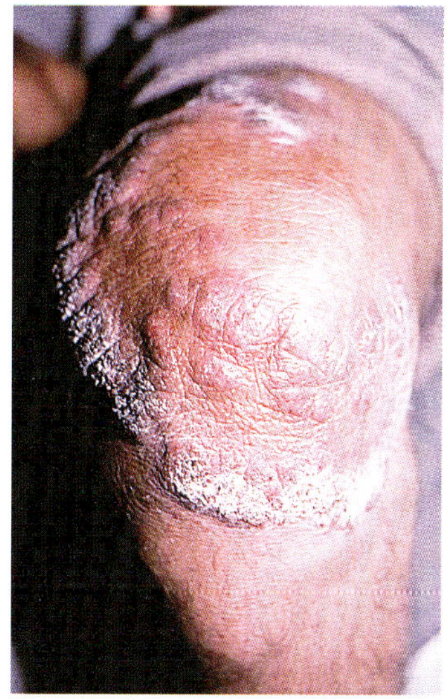

d

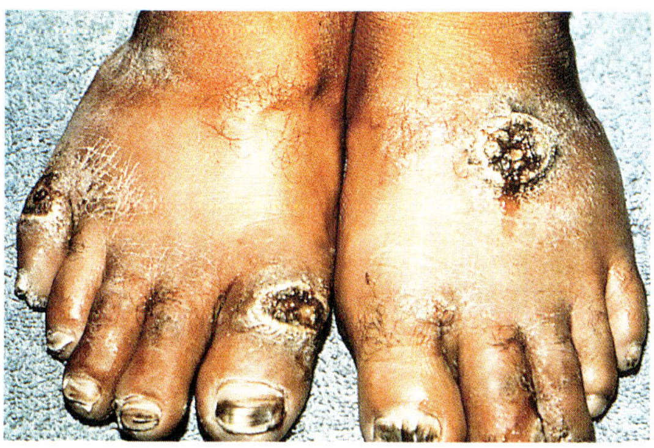

e

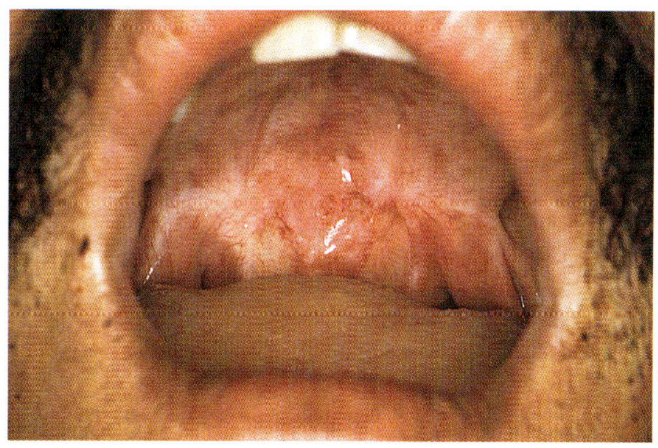

f

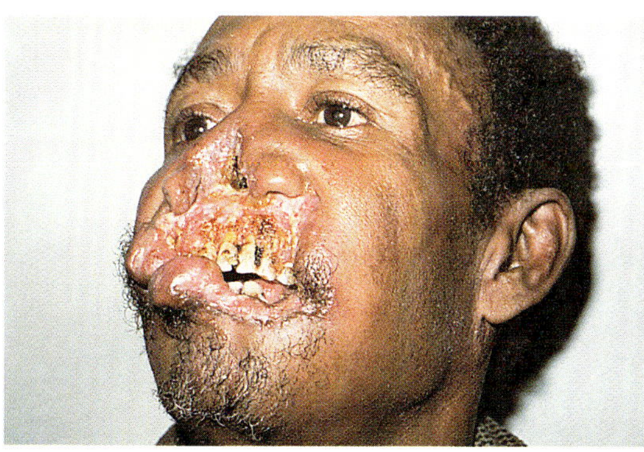

g

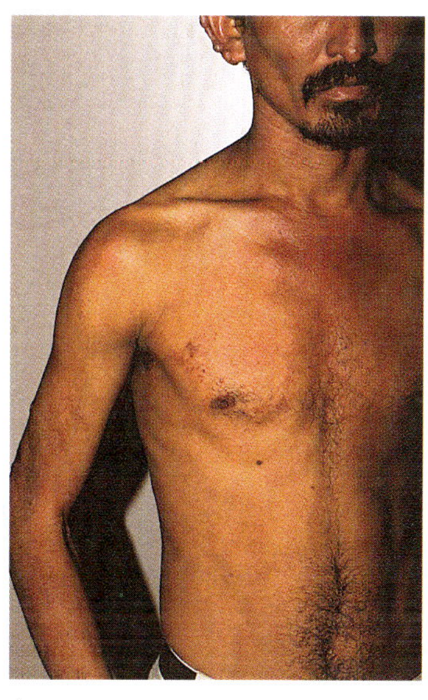

h

DIAGNOSIS

A presumptive diagnosis is made in endemic areas on the basis of clinical presentation. Confirmation is obtained by demonstrating leishmaniae on Giemsa-stained smears of lesions. *L. braziliensis* may be grown on NNN medium. The Montenegro intradermal test and lymphocyte transformation test are comparable to a tuberculin test for diagnostic purposes. Testing may also be done with a polymerase chain reaction.

DIFFERENTIAL DIAGNOSIS

Other granulomatous lesions may resemble leishmaniasis. Syphilis, mycobacterial diseases, deep mycoses, and even sarcoidosis also may resemble leishmaniasis.

TREATMENT

Many agents, ranging from cryotherapy to topical paromomycin, pentavalent antimonials, and macrolides to antifungal agents have been used with varying success.

SUGGESTED READINGS

Convit J, Ulrich M, Fernandez CT, et al. The clinical and immunological spectrum of American cutaneous leishmaniasis. Trans R Soc Med Hyg 1993;87:444–448.

de Brujin MH, Labrada LA, Smyth AJ, et al. A comparative study of diagnosis by the polymerase chain reaction and by current clinical methods using biopsies from Colombian patients with suspected leishmaniasis. Trop Med Parasitol 1993;44:201–207.

Frankenburg S, Klaus SN. Evaluation of a total lymphocyte proliferation assay as a diagnostic tool for cutaneous leishmaniasis. Trans R Soc Trop Med Hyg 1989;83:499–502.

Goihman-Yahr M. American mucocutaneous leishmaniasis. Dermatol Clin 1994;12:703–712.

Halmai-Stupar O, Arosemena-Sarkissian R, Paez E, et al. American cutaneous leishmaniasis: intermediate form. Int J Dermatol 1993;32:204–205.

Peters W, Killick-Kendrick R. The leishmaniases in biology and medicine. Orlando, FL: Academic Press, 1987:1–941.

Ramesh V, Misra RS, Saxena U, et al. Post-kala-azar dermal leishmaniasis: a clinical and therapeutic study. Int J Dermatol 1993;32:272–275.

Ramesh V, Mulcherjec A. Post-kala-azar dermal leishmaniasis. Int J Dermatol 1995;34:85–91.

FILARIASIS

Filariasis is a broad term implying infestation by filarial worms. A stricter definition limits it to those conditions due to Bancroftian and Malayan filariasis.

ETIOLOGY

Filariae (superfamily Filariodieae, class Nemathelminthes) are round worms resembling long white hairs. Species which afflict humans are characterized by (1) parasitism in the lymphatics or in the subcutaneous tissues, (2) liberation of active embryos (microfilariae) in the bloodstream or in the subcutaneous tissues, and (3) transmission of microfilariae by arthropod vectors (Table 13).

Table 13 Filarial Diseases

Filarial worm	Habitat of adults	Microfilariae	Vector/ transmission	Disease
Filaria bancrofti	lymphatics	blood, nocturnal	mosquitoes: *Anopheles, Culex*	filariasis
Wucheria malayi	lymphatics	blood, nocturnal	mosquitoes: *Mansonia*	filariasis
Onchocerca volvulus	subcutaneous tissue	subcutaneous tissue	gnats: *Simulium*	onchocerciasis
Loa-loa	subcutaneous tissue, blood, diurnal		horseflies: *Chrysops*	loiasis
Dracunculus	subcutaneous tissue	outside of skin	crustacean: *Cyclops medinensis* (contaminated water) (via ingestion)	dracunculiasis

CLINICAL PRESENTATION

Filariasis Common in tropical Africa (*F. bancfrofti*) and in the Far East (*W. malayi*). It begins with an asymptomatic period of 12 to 24 months or even many years. The active stage is characterized by recurrent episodes of acute lymphangitis of the legs, regional lymphadenitis, and orchitis. With progressive lymphatic obstruction, there is increasing edema, fibrosis, skin thickening, and, finally, elephantiasis (Figure 92a).

Onchocerciasis or nodular filariasis Encountered in central Africa and Central and South America. There is an incubation period of 1 year. The initial cutaneous changes are disseminated prurigo on the extensor surfaces of the extremities and the trunk (gale filarienne), which progress to lichenification and poikiloderma, and subcutaneous nodules on the extremities containing the encapsulated worm. Infestation of the anterior and posterior eye segments leads to blindness (Figure 92b).

Loiasis Found in west Africa. It is relatively benign and even asymptomatic. Skin lesions consist of transient, painless swelling (Calabar swelling) lasting a few days. The adult worm may then be seen creeping in the subcutaneous tissue or under the bulbar conjunctiva (Figure 92c).

Dracunculosis, or guinea worm infection Initially produces an anaphylactic reaction with urticaria, vomiting, diarrhea, and asthma. This is followed by a pustular eruption and ulceration through which the female worm reaches the skin to expel the microfilariae. A milky fluid is also discharged from the ulcer (Figure 92d).

DIAGNOSIS

Clinical findings may be supported by visualizing the worms (loiasis and dracontiasis) and demonstrating microfilariae in blood samples (filariasis and loiasis), in the ulcer, or in a superficial "exsanguineous" skin biopsy (onchocerciasis). Serodiagnosis and provocative in vivo testing with a single dose (50 to 100 mg) of diethylcarbamazine (Mazzoti test) assists in diagnosing onchocerciasis.

DIFFERENTIAL DIAGNOSIS

Numerous pyogenic and eczematous reactions can be confused with these infestations.

TREATMENT

Diethylcarbamazine, 6 mg/kg for 12 days, and ivermetin, 150 gm/kg, may be used, along with symptomatic treatment and microbial coverage for secondary infection.

SUGGESTED READINGS

Evans DB, Gelband H, Vlassoff C. Social and economic factors and the control of lymphatics. Acta Trop (Basel) 1993;53:1–26.

Glickman LT, Magnaval JF. Zoonotic roundworm infections. Infect Dis Clin North Am 1993;7:717–732.

Ottesen EA. Filarial infections. Infect Dis Clin North Am 1993;7:619–633.

Routh HB. Elephantiasis. Int J Dermatol 1992;31:845–855.

Routh HB, Bhowmik KR. Filariasis. Dermatol Clin 1994;12:719–728.

Storey DM. Filariasis: nutritional interactions in human and animal hosts. Parasitology 1993;107(suppl):S147–158.

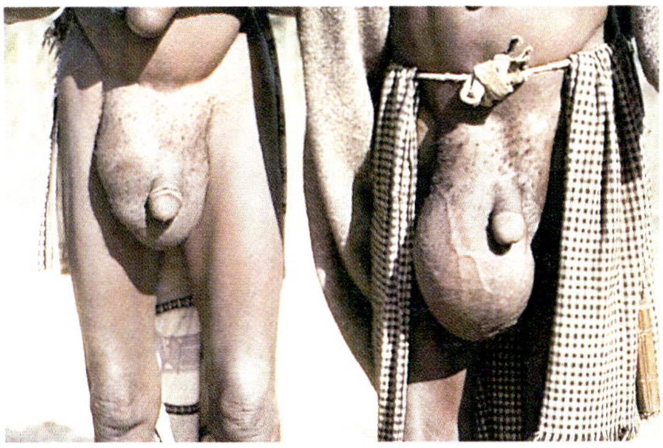

a

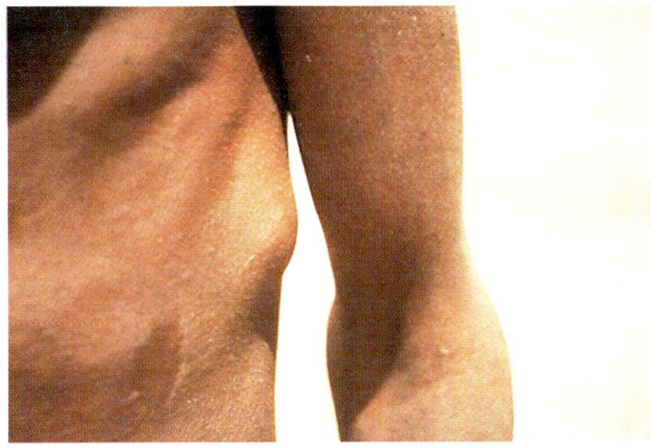

b

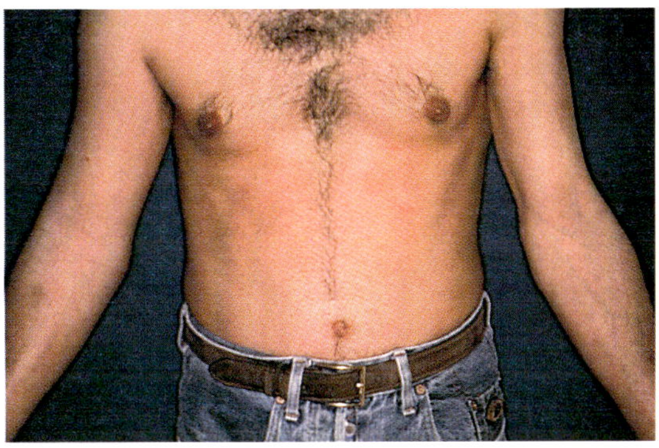

c

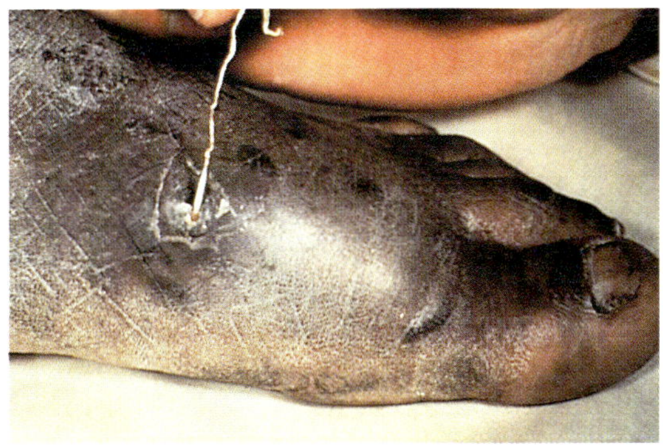

d

Figure 92
(a) Filariasis eventually leads to elephantiasis. (Courtesy of Michel Larivière, MD, Paris, France.) (b) Onchocerciasis develops into an atrophic hypopigmented dermatitis. (c) Loiasis is characterized by red nodules, often confluent, known as Calabar swellings. (Courtesy of Michel Larivière, MD, Paris, France.) (d) Dracunculiasis may be diagnosed by extracting the worm. (Courtesy of Michel Larivière, MD, Paris, France.)

Ancylostomiasis

Ancylostomiasis includes hookworm disease and creeping eruption. These conditions, preponderant in the tropics, can be found anywhere in the world.

ETIOLOGY

The hookworms *Ancylostoma* are small (up to 10 nm), intestinal nematodes. The eggs are spread by feces in the soil, in which the larvae hatch. Ground itch is caused by *Ancylostoma duodenale* and *Necator americanus*, when they penetrate the skin. Spread is hematogenous. Creeping eruption is caused by the penetration of the incompletely developed larvae of the zoophilic *A. braziliense*.

CLINICAL PRESENTATION

Ground itch Manifested by pruritic, erythematous urticarial to papulovesicular lesions, often on the feet. When the hookworm penetrates to the intestinal tract, there may be such systemic signs as weight loss, anemia, dyspnea, myalgia, and abdominal pains (Figure 93a).

Cutaneous larva migrans (creeping eruption) Characterized by an intensely pruritic eruption at the site of penetration of larvae. As the worm moves in the skin, up to 2 to 5 cm daily, strange flesh-colored to red bands appear. Spontaneous healing can occur within 2 months (Figure 93b).

DIAGNOSIS

Clinical manifestations may be substantiated by finding the eggs and the worms.

DIFFERENTIAL DIAGNOSIS

Contact dermatitis, dermatophytosis, and pyodermas may have similar presentations.

TREATMENT

Hookworm infection requires systemic administration of thiabendazole (25 mg/kg) for 5 days, pirantel (10 mg/kg) in a single dose, or albendazole (200 mg) in a single dose. Creeping eruption may be treated by cryosurgery, with thiabendazole cream 15% applied three times daily for several days.

SUGGESTED READINGS

Amer M. Antiparasitic therapy. In: Parish LC, Millikan LE, Amer M, et al, eds. Global Dermatology. New York: Springer-Verlag, 1994:331–339.

Davis HD, Sakuls P, Keystone JS. Creeping eruption: a review of clinical presentation and management of 60 cases presenting to a tropical disease unit. Arch Dermatol 1993;129:588–591.

Guilman RH. Hookworm disease: host pathogen biology. Rev Infect Dis 1982;4:824–835.

Katz M, Despommier DD, Gwadz RW. Parasitic diseases. New York: Springer-Verlag, 1986:16–21.

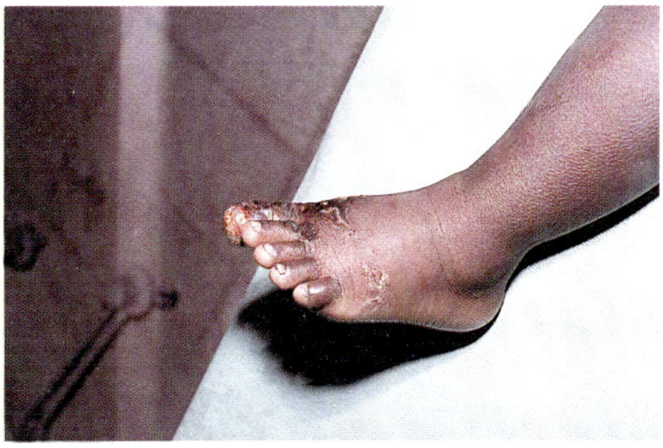

a

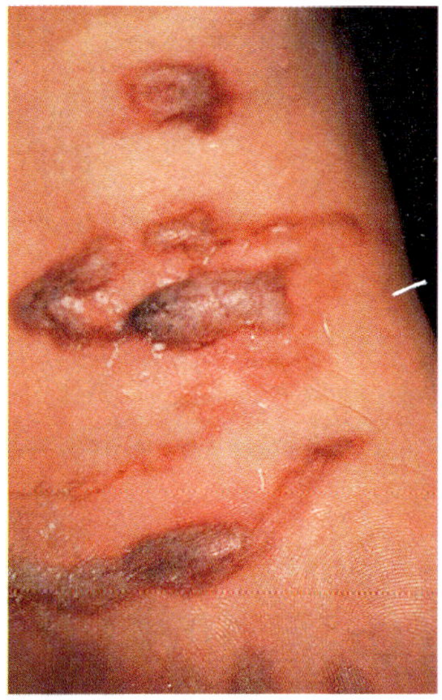

b

Figurc 93
(a) Ground itch is characterized by crusting and erosions on the foot. (Courtesy of Bassirou Ndiaye, MD, Dakar, Senegal.) (b) Cutaneous larva migrans may have bullae as well as red serpiginous lesions. (Courtesy of Michel Larivière, MD, Paris, France.)

Schistosomiasis

Schistosomiasis, also known as *bilharziasis*, is a worldwide health problem affecting approximately 200 million people.

ETIOLOGY

Schistosomiasis is caused by blood flukes or flat worms, known as *Schistosoma mansoni* and *S. haematobium,* which are intestinal parasites, and *S. japonica,* which is an urinary tract parasite. The eggs excreted by the worms undergo transformation into active larvae (cercariae) in the intermediate host (molluscs) on contact with water. The cercariae penetrate the skin, provoking cercarial dermatitis, and move on to the bloodstream. Late cutaneous schistosomiasis occurs when adult worms deposit their eggs in the dermis.

CLINICAL PRESENTATION

Cercarial dermatitis, or swimmer's itch Develops 15 to 30 minutes after contact with water. There are pruritic, pin-point red macules, urticaria, and even vesicles at the site of penetration of the cercariae. The zoophilic form is more pronounced. Lesions usually resolve within 1 to 3 weeks but leave residual hypo- and hyperpigmentation (Figure 94a).

Late cutaneous schistosomiasis, or bilharziasis cutanea tarda Presents with soft, nontender, vegetating papules and nodules that may suppurate and ulcerate. The lesions are found on the genitalia and perianal areas, although occasionally some appear on the trunk. Rarely, there may be malignant transformation (Figure 94b).

Schistosomides, or bilharzides May occur in the invasive stage or in the course of visceral schistosomiasis. There are pruritic, urticarial, edematous, and purplish lesions.

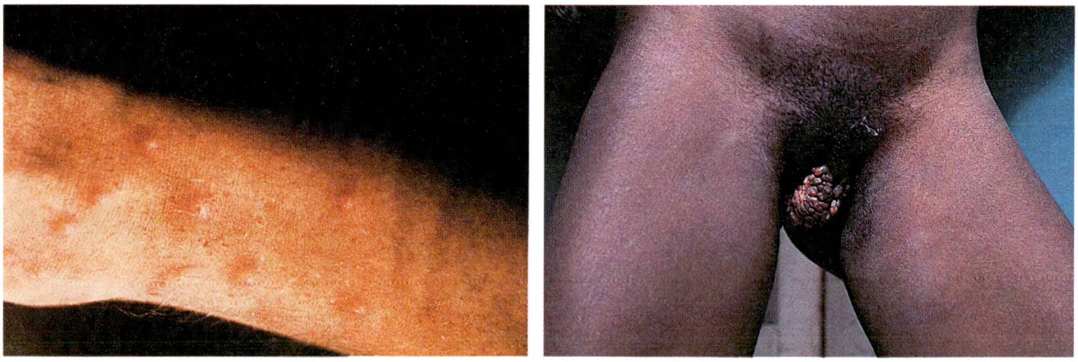

a b

Figure 94
(a) Cercarial dermatitis may present as itchy red nodules. (Courtesy of Wolfram Höffler, MD, Tübingen, Germany.) (b) Late cutaneous schistosomiasis is characterized by vegetative nodules on the scrotum. (Courtesy of Bassirou Ndiaye, MD, Dakar, Senegal.)

DIAGNOSIS

Swimmer's itch is diagnosed by the chronologic relationship between the eruption and the contact with open waters. Late cutaneous schistosomiasis is presumed in endemic areas and confirmed by finding the eggs in feces, urine, or biopsies from the rectal mucosa or the skin.

DIFFERENTIAL DIAGNOSIS

Contact dermatitis and granulomatous infections may be confused with these infestations.

TREATMENT

Cercarial dermatitis is treated effectively with thiabendazole (50 mg/kg) for 1 to 2 days or praziquantel (25 mg/kg) in a single dose. The latter is also effective in *S. japonica* visceral infection. *S. haematobium* and *S. mansoni* are treated with metrifonate (7.5 mg/kg), repeated twice at biweekly intervals, or with oxamniquine (20 mg/kg) in a single dose.

SUGGESTED READINGS

Amer M. Cutaneous schistosomiasis. Dermatol Clin 1994;12:713–718.

González E. Schistosomiasis: hope for a vaccine. J Clin Dermatol 1994;1 (May/June): 33–34.

Katz M, Despommier DD, Gwadz RW. Parasitic diseases. New York: Springer-Verlag, 1986:94–105.

Scott JA, Davidson RN, Moody AH, et al. Diagnosing multiple parasitic infections: trypanosomiasis, loiasis and schistosomiasis in a single case. Scand J Infect Dis 1991;23:777–780.

INDEX

V

W

Y